MORE PRAISE FOR *YOUR HANDS CAN HEAL YOU*

"*Your Hands Can Heal You* is an incredibly powerful text for working with energy through simple, effective healing exercises. Master Co and Dr. Robins clearly describe the life force known as "prana" and provide practical instructions for directing and managing your pranic energy in all aspects of your life and health. This book is more than brilliant—it is essential for all readers who value the quality of their health."

—*Caroline Myss, author,* Sacred Contracts *and* Anatomy of the Spirit

"The authors have transformed ancient Eastern healing traditions into digestible food for thought for the Western mind. This wonderful interpretation allows healers from all walks of life to reengage these fascinating techniques."

—*Mehmet Oz, M.D., co-founder, Complementary Care Center at New York's Columbia-Presbyterian Hospital, and author,* Healing from the Heart

"In one of my darkest hours, I discovered that Stephen Co is a masterful and loving healing agent! What he taught me to do with my hands was a gift. What he reminded me that I had the power to do was a blessing!"

—*Iyanla Vanzant, author,* One Day My Soul Just Opened Up

"Healing is one of the greatest arts. My friend Stephen is a master healer and teacher. Use his brilliance to heal yourself, others and our world."

—*Mark Victor Hansen, co-creator, No. 1 New York Times bestselling series*
Chicken Soup for the Soul®

"*Your Hands Can Heal You* is a fascinating and practical study of an ancient and natural healing system. I found it captivating."

—*Francis Ford Coppola, Academy Award Winning Director of* The Godfather Trilogy

"Master Stephen Co is an extraordinary, gentle man whose work expands one's understanding of the mysterious workings of the human body. In a seemingly egoless way, he shares his phenomenal knowledge and talent so that others can benefit from all he has discovered. I admire him very much."

—*Mary Steenburgen, actress, producer, writer*

"This book not only offers a practical, enjoyable guide to working with your own health and transformation, it is a doorway to the world of subtle energy."

—*Rudolph Ballentine, M.D., author,* Radical Healing

"*Your Hands Can Heal You* offers an elegantly simple guide to using your own natural spiritual resources to enhance your flow of vibrant energy."

—*Gay Hendricks, Ph.D., author,*
Conscious Loving *and* Achieving Vibrance

"Eighty-five percent of illnesses are not optimally treatable with drugs or surgery. For those individuals, *Your Hands Can Heal You* offers one of the best self-healing approaches I have seen."

—*C. Norman Shealy, M.D., Ph.D., president, Holistic Institutes of Health*

"Pranic Healing techniques, especially the Meditation on Twin Hearts, help me to be more present in daily life and have had a powerful, positive effect on my wife and me. After a Pranic Healing treatment, Julie says that my voice sounds as if I had received a full body massage. To me it's an internal massage. I sleep better and my emotional clarity is more grounded. I still feel life's ups and downs but with Pranic Healing and meditation, I feel that I don't have to stay in those negative states of emotion for a long time. I have the freedom to let go of unhelpful emotions."

—*Tom Skerritt, actor, producer, writer*

"Master Co is one of the most interesting, intriguing healers that I have ever had the honor of being touched by. With this book he shows us how to access the power to heal that has always been and will always be within us. I adore him."

—*Melanie Griffith, actress, producer, writer*

"I used to drive three hours to spend time with Master Co. Thank God he's written this book. His brilliance and generosity have given us all the gift of self-healing. Plus, the commute is much easier."

—*Ted Danson, Emmy Award and Golden Globe Award–Winning actor and producer*

"As a television reporter, I have hundreds of healing techniques and so-called miracle cures cross my desk. The energy remedies you are about to read in *Your Hands Can Heal You* are the real deal. After we aired a news story on Master Stephen Co, Dr. Eric Robins, and Pranic Healing, my mailbox overflowed with thank-you letters from viewers who learned and were helped by the technique. Their book contains so much valuable information."

—*Jennifer Sabih, CBS News*

"*Your Hands Can Heal You* is a wonderful, exciting new approach to healing. A self-help guide to healing thyself by combining and synthesizing basic approaches to many healing modalities, with the unique experiential techniques of Pranic Healing. A must-read for every person interested in the art of healing."

—*Barry Hirsch J.D., Premier Entertainment Industry Attorney*

"After a Pranic Healing, your mind feels clearer, a sense of peacefulness, being in oneness with the world. Renewed enthusiasm and confidence."

—*Marilyn Ghigliotti, actress*

"Through his personal sessions, classes, and now through his writings, Master Co's paradigm-shifting model goes right to the heart of healing: we are our healing practitioners working directly in the laboratory of consciousness with prana, the Divine Life Force that maintains our very existence. More personally, Master Co is a man of integrity, wisdom, and power."

—*Revevend Michael Beckwith, Founder and Spiritual Director,*
The Agape International Spiritual Center

YOUR HANDS CAN HEAL YOU

Pranic Healing Energy
Remedies to Boost
Vitality and Speed Recovery
from Common Health Problems

by Master Stephen Co and Eric B. Robins, M.D.
with John Merryman

ATRIA PAPERBACK
New York • London • Toronto • Sydney • New Delhi

ATRIA PAPERBACK
A Division of Simon & Schuster, Inc.
1230 Avenue of the Americas
New York, NY 10020

First Atria Paperback edition August 2013

ATRIA PAPERBACK and colophon are trademarks of
Simon & Schuster Inc.

For information regarding special discounts for bulk purchases,
please contact Simon & Schuster Special Sales
at 1-866-506-1949 or business@simonandschuster.com.

The Simon & Schuster Speakers Bureau can bring authors to your
live event. For more information or to book an event, contact
Simon & Schuster Speakers Bureau at 1-866-248-3049 or visit our
website at www.simonspeakers.com.

Manufactured in the United States of America

30 29 28 27 26 25

Library of Congress Cataloging-in-Publication Data

Co, Stephen.
   Your hands can heal you : pranic healing energy remedies to boost
vitality and speed recovery from common health problems /
by Stephen Co and Eric B. Robins, with John Merryman.
      p. cm.
   Includes bibliographical references and index.
   1. Healing. 2. Vital force. 3. Mental healing. I. Robins, Eric B.
   II. Merryman, John. III. Title.

RZ401 .C597 2002

615.8'51—dc21   2002029949

ISBN 978-0-7432-3562-4
ISBN 978-0-7432-4305-6 (pbk)
ISBN 978-1-4165-9594-6 (ebook)

To Grandmaster Choa Kok Sui:

May this book be instrumental in rapidly disseminating your

priceless teachings to uplift humanity.

ACKNOWLEDGMENTS

My deepest thanks to:

Divine Providence and the Great Ones, whose boundless love and blessings make everything possible.

First and foremost, my beloved and respected Teacher, Grandmaster Choa Kok Sui, for allowing us to write this book using materials and teaching from his Pranic Self-Healing Course; from his book, *Miracles Through Pranic Healing*; and from many of his other private teachings and notes never before made available to the general public. I am especially grateful for his love, priceless teachings, blessings, patience, and for his giving me the opportunity to serve.

All my other teachers for my early years of learning and nurturing.

My parents, for bringing me into this world and for the sacrifices they have made to give me a good education and upbringing.

My wife, Daphne, and my two jewels, Genevie and Helena, for their continuous support and understanding and especially for the sacrifices they have made to bring me to the path of service.

Dr. Eric Robins and John Merryman, for their expertise, support, and dedication. All those who helped us get the book out: our editor, Leslie Meredith, for her invaluable industry expertise and dedication to making sure the book was "just right"; Dorothy Robinson, for being super supportive in getting all the details taken care of perfectly; Amy Heller, for her untiring publicity support; our agent, Mary Tahan, and also Stedman Mays, from Clausen, Mays & Tahan, for working so hard to get us the right publisher; our publicist, Arielle Ford, and her great crew, Katherine and Cameron, for their tireless promotion efforts; and Marv Wolf, for his insightful editorial comments on the manuscript.

Karla Alvarez, for her untiring assistance in moving the Pranic Healing mission forward.

Ximena Valencia, for the wonderful artwork, and Chet Smith, for the excellent photography.

The entire Pranic Healing family, for their unending dedication to spreading these priceless teachings to alleviate the suffering of humanity.

Countless others not mentioned, for their valuable suggestions and contributions.

—*Master Stephen Co*

* * *

I have many people to thank for helping this book reach fruition. First and foremost, a thank-you to Grandmaster Choa Kok Sui for allowing us to write this book using his own research, materials, and teachings. I feel personally blessed that he has given us so much proprietary material to share with a much wider audience. Grandmaster Choa has patiently taken me under his wing as a student, and for that I am much indebted. Also a thank-you to John Merryman, who put our thoughts, words, and speeches into writing. While Grandmaster Choa provided the inspiration for this book, John provided the perspiration.

I could not have written this book without the unfailing love and support of my wife, Linda, and son, Jonah. They have truly been the "power behind the power" (as Master Choa is fond of saying). A thanks also goes out to my parents for the excellent job they did in raising me, and particularly to my father, who used to make me sit with him while he read me long stories of great yogis.

I have had many teachers in the mind/body/energy field. Foremost among these have been Master Stephen Co, Tad James, Cal Banyan, Steve Parkhill, and Gay Hendricks, Ph.D. Kudos go to Bob Coffman, my bioenergetic therapist, who has definitely shown me the way to self-love. Thanks also to Tom Vandergast, M.D., my chief of urology, who has been one of my biggest supporters and fans, and whose support has been vital in my helping to bring these types of teachings into the mainstream medical community.

A heartfelt thanks and a hug to Mary Tahan, our agent; Leslie Meredith, our editor at the Free Press; and Arielle Ford, our publicist. Additional thanks to Marv Wolf for his editorial review and comments.

Last, to Jim Sorden and Daniel O'Hara, both of whom have been close friends in the Pranic Healing family. Jim is the person I go to when I need a healing, and Dan is someone who, when professional sports establishments find out the efficacy of Pranic Healing for their injured players, will be in tremendous demand.

—*Eric B. Robins, M.D.*

CONTENTS

FOREWORD by Grandmaster Choa Kok Sui   xiii

INTRODUCTION by Eric B. Robins, M.D.   1

    Note on Nomenclature   6

PART I – HOW YOUR BODY AND MIND WORK

CHAPTER 1:   You're Wired for Healing —Your Energetic Anatomy   9

CHAPTER 2:   The True Nature of Your Mind—How It Protects You and Hurts You   31

PART II – THE SIX STEPS TO SELF-HEALING

STEP 1: Clearing Negative Emotions and Limiting Beliefs

CHAPTER 3:   All Clear!—Removing Emotionally Based Energetic Blockages   45

STEP 2: Pranic Breathing

CHAPTER 4:   Take a Deep Breath—Pranic Breathing   62

STEP 3: Energy Manipulation

CHAPTER 5:   Hands Up! Scanning—Hand Sensitivity
and General Scanning   82

CHAPTER 6:   Hands Up! More Scanning—Specific Scanning and Interpreting Results   97

CHAPTER 7:   Out With the Old—Sweeping Away Congested Energy,
             Cleaning Your Aura   111

CHAPTER 8:   Pump It Up—Energizing Areas of Depletion   142

CHAPTER 9:   Rainbow Power—Using Colors   155

             STEP 4: Energetic Hygiene
CHAPTER 10: Keep It Clean—The Importance of Energetic Hygiene   177

             STEP 5: Meditation
CHAPTER 11: Easy Ways to Put Your Mind at Ease—Meditations
             for Peace and Stillness   199

             STEP 6: Energy-Generation Exercises
CHAPTER 12: Plugging In, Charging Up—Two Powerful Energy-Generation Exercises   220

PART III – STAYING ENERGIZED AND HEALTHY

CHAPTER 13: A Self-Healing Guide—Energetic Solutions to 24 Common
             Health Problems   245

CHAPTER 14: Prescription for Greater Energy and Better Health—
             The *Your Hands Can Heal You* Daily Routine   262

PART IV – BEYOND PHYSICAL HEALTH

CHAPTER 15: You've Got Soul—Physical Health, Spiritual Development, and Beyond . . .   267

             Sources and Notes   284
             For Further Reference   287
             Index   293

FOREWORD

Today more than ever, we all have a tremendous need for rapid, effective methods of balancing the material and spiritual aspects of our life. At the same time, we are experiencing a mass awakening of consciousness, which has created in many people a need to seek spiritual solutions to everyday life situations, such as stress, relationships, success, failure, and perhaps most of all, health.

I believe this book will greatly help to meet these needs.

It presents a simple, effective way to increase your health and personal energy through working at deeper emotional and energetic levels of reality, where you can increase, control, and direct your personal supply of prana, the universal life force that your body uses for healing.

When you gain control over your personal health, you increase your ability to live a full life and experience all this world has to offer. But learning how to heal your aches, pains, and illnesses is really just the beginning of your healing journey, for as you enter this path, your consciousness will be stirred to recognize greater truths. The most important of these is that we are all parts of a larger whole, a bioenergetic system that represents the sum total of the energy of each of us. As a result, we are interdependent upon one another for energy— and for life. This interdependence means that the choices we make in our lives have an effect—physically and energetically—on everyone around us. When we take steps to heal ourselves, we contribute positive emotions and energy to that system; we heal the world.

That is the ultimate goal of Pranic Healing.

So as you begin your study of these simple, effective healing techniques, I offer my love, blessings, and hopes that you achieve all your personal self-healing goals. But I also hope that you become aware of the important role you play in increasing the health and energy of the world in which we live and work, and that you use the teachings in this book to that end as well.

With love and blessings, Grandmaster Choa Kok Sui

DISCLAIMER

This publication contains the opinions and ideas of its authors. It is intended to provide helpful and informative material on the subjects it addresses. It is sold with the understanding that the author and publisher are not engaged in rendering medical, health, or any other kind of personal professional services in the book. The reader should consult his or her medical, health, or other competent professional before adopting any of the suggestions in this book or drawing inferences from it.

The author and publisher specifically disclaim all responsibility for any liability, loss, or risk, personal or otherwise, that is incurred as a consequence, directly or indirectly, of the use and application of any of the contents of this book.

The names and characteristics of some individuals in this book have been changed.

YOUR HANDS
CAN
HEAL YOU

INTRODUCTION:
Your Hands Can Heal You

I n the often irreverent language of the operating room, James was "circling the drain." Quite simply, he was going to die. A 41-year-old man who had been hospitalized for gall bladder surgery in the Los Angeles medical center where I worked, James had developed a host of serious postoperative complications: yeast sepsis (a blood infection fatal 70 percent of the time), a blood clot in the lung (fatal nearly 60 percent of the time), and multiple enterocutaneous fistulae (openings in his abdominal wall through which intestinal fluid was leaking). In addition, he had daily fever spikes of up to 104 degrees, constant nausea, and vomiting.

Three months earlier I had taken a class called "Introduction to Pranic Healing," an energy medicine system that teaches people to manipulate the body's prana, or vital force, to facilitate healing. I remembered vividly our instructor's confidence in the system. Master Pranic Healer Stephen Co, one of the world's top practitioners, frequently urged us to "do the practice and look for the results; don't take my word for it that it works."

I had practiced and had produced a few results, but nothing spectacular. But I had used the system only to relax some of my patients who were nervous, stressed, or anxious. I had never tried it on anyone with a substantial health problem. After watching James languishing in the intensive care unit for months, though, and knowing that his surgeon held little hope for his survival, I decided to put Pranic Healing to a real test. I asked James' surgeon if I could try "something different" with his patient; he agreed.

At that time I was making a name for myself around the hospital as an advocate for alternative healing methods alongside traditional Western scientific medicine. To be sure, my advocacy did not sit well with some of my colleagues. Although some physicians accept alternative and complementary medical treatments today, many remain skeptical. But being a board-certified urologist and surgeon with a reputation for a rigorously scientific approach to diagnosis and treatment—and having the backing of an open-minded department chief—I knew that I had the support to promote my beliefs.

If some of my more progressive physician colleagues had peeked through the curtains

I drew around James' bed as I began his treatment, however, they might have wondered if I weren't trying something a little *too* different. They would have seen me standing a few feet away from James, moving my hands swiftly and silently in the air around his illness-ravaged body. Some of the movements I made were smooth and circular; others were sharp and angular. Every so often, I moistened my hands with a spray bottle filled with alcohol lightly scented with lavender. I waved my arms around James like this for almost 30 minutes.

I must confess that as I left James' bedside, I wasn't sure what type of results I had produced. I knew, however, that I had kept an open mind and a positive attitude, and that I had followed the instructions I had learned in the Pranic Healing class.

The next day James' fever and nausea were gone. The scientist in me, of course, wondered if it had been some type of spontaneous remission, because such things occasionally happen. Outwardly, I was cool and detached, the professional physician. Inside, though, I was tremendously excited; I couldn't help but think that Pranic Healing did work. I also couldn't wait to get back and apply another treatment. To make a long story short, after one week of daily Pranic Healing treatments, James' pulse rate and pulmonary function stabilized. After two more weeks of Pranic Healing treatments, he strengthened visibly. Within a month, he was healthy enough to undergo a final surgery to repair his fistulae. Defying the predictions of his physicians, James made a full recovery. Today, nearly three years later, he stops by my office occasionally just to say hello.

A miracle? To those who hold a strictly traditional Western view of medical science, perhaps, but not to me. Not now. Not after what I've seen accomplished with Pranic Healing.

Here's an even more dramatic example of Pranic Healing, performed by Master Stephen Co. It was featured on a syndicated television program, but the following text is taken directly from a signed and dated testimonial by the woman whom Master Co treated:

Four years ago in March 1992, I was diagnosed with a platelet disorder, hypercoagulable state, which left me legally blind in my left eye from a central retinal vein occlusion. I was placed on many different medications: blood thinners, steroids, and blood pressure sedatives. Plus, I had had nine laser and cryonics surgeries on my eye. Two and a half months ago, after visiting you and receiving Pranic Healing, not only could I see clearly out of my left eye, but I also had my blood checked the following Monday at the hematologist's office, and there was no indication of the blood clotting disorder. My bleeding was normal. I have been off all medication for almost three months. I am still seeing clearly out of my left eye, and I feel normal for the first time in years. You've given me hope and happiness that now I, too, can have a future free of pain and confusion and hardship.

—JILL SCHWARTZ, LOS ANGELES

Jill Schwartz's doctors at UCLA Medical Center verified that her hypercoagulable state was gone. Here are some other examples of ordinary people who used Pranic Healing to help themselves heal simple, complex, and even life-threatening health problems. In each case, the text is taken directly from signed and dated statements. The colors to which they refer are types of energy or prana that you learn to use in Pranic Healing. "Sweeping," "cleansing," and "energizing" are other Pranic Healing techniques.

I do want to emphasize, however, that should you suffer any of these accidents or illnesses, you should seek professional medical help immediately.

I work as a repair technician for Motorola, Inc., in the cellular phone division. The printed circuit boards are surface mount boards. To remove components, we use a 600-watt heat gun designed to strip linoleum off floors. Its nose is a metal piece about 4 inches long. One morning, my bench partner used the heat gun and placed it (still hot) on my bench while I was concentrating on tracing a signal on the circuit board before me. It toppled over and landed squarely on the top of my right hand. My initial reaction was shock. Once I looked at my hand and saw the entire surface turn red and start to bubble up, I snapped into action. I immediately began to sweep with whitish-green. The pain began to set in. It was very intense. I then recalled the effects of blue. I energized the hand with whitish-blue to numb the pain. . . . I alternated whitish-green with whitish-orange. I did continual sweeping for about an hour. I saw the size of the welt decrease. This encouraged me to continue. As the day went on, word spread about what had happened. People looked on in disbelief. In four hours, the size was reduced to a half-inch. Everyone kept telling me I'd get a blister and be scarred for life. I continued to ignore them and kept sweeping my hand throughout the day. I felt no pain, and the wound never blistered. Once I got home, there was a small mark on the surface of my right hand. I continued to sweep with whitish-orange, then I energized with whitish-red and a touch of whitish-yellow. Today my hand looks like nothing ever happened. Since I have learned Pranic Healing, any cut or bruise never fully manifests on my body. I use it on pimples and cold sores upon the start of a breakout, and in a few minutes they disappear.

—ELIZABETH SEDENO, CHICAGO

On Friday, May 12, 2000, at approximately 8:12 A.M., the symptoms began with a severe headache. [When] the pain spread into my neck, I became very aware that there was a good possibility that I was having a stroke. I called for an ambulance. As the pain intensified, a strange calm came over me, which allowed me to recall self-healing techniques taught by Master Co. While the excruciating pain made it most difficult to concentrate, it did not make it impossible to make a conscious decision to ask for and seek divine intervention. During my prayer for help, the memory of Pranic Healing class was given back to me . . . [and] a brilliant white shaft of light appeared on my crown chakra. It was transparent, yet dense in appearance and form. If I were to guess, it was approximately 14 inches in diameter. It remained attached to my body throughout my crisis.

I was transferred from a local emergency room and became an ICU patient at a trauma hospital. The diagnosis was that I had suffered a cerebral aneurysm. The location was in the center of my brain. For the next three days, I meditated on healing the aneurysm by bathing the area in the healing white light. While visualizing the white light coming from my fingers, I also visualized stroking the brain. These two mental activities became my main objective throughout my stay at the hospital. By the fourth day of my stay in ICU, after reviewing the third CAT scan, one of the doctors said, "If I didn't know better, this looks as if I'd already performed the surgery!" On day number five in ICU, my nurse became concerned because of the extremely high level of potassium in my system. I have since learned that potassium guards against stroke. The more you have in the system, the greater the protection against stroke. Finally, I went from high-risk intensive care to home in eight days. I did not require surgery. Once home, I took salt baths one to two times a day for the first three days. After that, two salt baths a day for a week. It has been 13 months since my illness with no recurring symptoms.

—CYNTHIA A. BORMAN, HOMEWOOD, ILLINOIS

While driving a wooden stake into the ground, a portion (about ⅛ inch) broke off and was driven into my hand. Pliers were required to remove the piece. Only soap and water were used on [the wound]. I immediately began Pranic Healing and all bleeding stopped. Within a half-hour, all pain and swelling was diminished. Two days later a thick scab had formed, and healing was almost complete. This occurred three days ago, and the wound is almost healed. Also, while spray-painting outdoors, a gust of wind blew the paint onto my face and into my eyes. Severe burning began in the eyes and on the eyelids. Even though I washed out my eyes with water, the next day, my eyes were swollen and quite painful. I began Pranic Healing. Relief began within 10 to 30 minutes. [I achieved] complete healing after two hours. No red remained in the eyes. All pain and swelling were totally gone. I have had no lingering problem with my eyes or eyelids since that procedure. In fact, the chronic eye irritation from crusted eyelids has been greatly improved as well!

—MAUREEN KELLEHER, ST. LOUIS

After hearing about numerous similar Pranic Healing success stories and after seeing the system work so well with my own patients, I became eager to share this information—and particularly the self-healing application—with more people. Coincidentally, Master Stephen Co had been considering different ways to reach the many people interested in learning Pranic Healing but who weren't able to attend a seminar. With the blessings and approval of Grandmaster Choa Kok Sui, the creator of the Pranic Healing system, we began to develop the program that has become the book you now hold in your hands.

We started with the basic Pranic Healing curriculum taught in Pranic Healing workshops and refocused it more specifically on self-healing. We added a number of new exercises and techniques never before seen in print or revealed outside Grandmaster Choa's classes. Then we enhanced the material further with several powerful, complementary, energy medicine practices from other disciplines. The result is *Your Hands Can Heal You*, an easy-to-follow program that enables you to increase your own personal supply of vital force or prana and then direct it for self-healing, just as the people in the testimonials did.

The testimonials here are remarkable but not unique. These people did not have any special healing gift, aptitude, or training before they learned Pranic Healing. They simply kept an open mind, followed the step-by-step instructions, practiced them, and applied them as needed.

For you to be successful at self-healing, all you need do is observe that same routine: Keep an open mind, perform the routine and exercises in this book as they are described, and practice regularly so that you are ready to use them when you need to.

If you follow this routine, you will realize what thousands of people who have learned Pranic Healing have discovered: Your hands *can* heal you.

—ERIC B. ROBINS, M.D., LOS ANGELES

NOTE ON NOMENCLATURE

On the terms "Grandmaster" and "Master": "Grandmaster" and "master" are popularly accepted terms in traditional Oriental culture and are used in many practices or systems that have their origin in the East (e.g., yoga, martial arts, etc.) to designate one who has achieved an exceptionally high level of training and accomplishment. These are secular titles, and their use in this book carries no connotation—religious, political, or otherwise—outside the context of Pranic Healing and Grandmaster Choa's teachings.

All illustrations, exercises, tables, and photographs are identified by chapter number, a dash, and then either a number, letter, or Roman numeral.

Illustrations, or figures, are indicated with numbers. Examples: Figure 4–2, Figure 7–1.

Exercises are indicated with capital letters. Examples: Exercise 4–A, Exercise 12–A.

Tables are indicated with capital Roman numerals. Examples: Table 1–I, Table 3–II.

Photographs are indicated with lower case letters. Examples: Photo 4–c, Photo 12–d.

Part I

How Your Body and Mind Work

CHAPTER 1

You're Wired
For Healing—Your
Energetic Anatomy

"During one of his healing sessions, Grandmaster Choa Kok Sui was working on a person who was a heavy drinker, though the person did not offer this information before the healing. Grandmaster Choa found a significant imbalance in this man's energy body—specifically in his liver—and told him that he should see a physician as soon as possible. The man went to the doctor and had a blood test, but the results indicated that his liver was fine. He received no medical treatment. Several months later, however, he developed severe pain in his liver. Tests at that time showed that he had hepatitis. We tell this story to students to demonstrate that we have an energetic anatomy *just as we have a physical anatomy, and to illustrate that illnesses manifest in your energy body (also called your energetic anatomy) before they appear in the physical body."*

—MASTER STEPHEN CO

Your body already heals itself.

You may take antibiotics to combat infections, dose yourself with aspirin to reduce pain, get a cast on a broken wrist, or even have your appendix removed by a surgeon, but drugs and medical procedures themselves don't "heal" you. They reduce inflammation, battle bacteria, or in the case of a cast or operation, make proper healing possible. But your body heals itself. And it does it magnificently. Through some process that we don't fully understand, your body has the amazing, innate ability to repair itself.

Medical science can explain the neurological and biochemical responses involved in healing a cut finger: The nerves carry the pain message to your brain to indicate a problem; white blood cells rush to the area to combat dirt or germs; platelets clot the blood and begin forming a scab; and the skin cells grow back underneath the scab. But medical science does not know how the body knows how to do this, and it doesn't know what force powers this healing process.

We know intuitively that there must be a consciousness behind this self-healing ability, one that knows how to work in the same way that our body knows how to breathe without our having to command our lungs to inhale and exhale. We have a storehouse of energy that our body uses for healing. Otherwise, white blood cells wouldn't be able to multiply and carry away infection and inflammation from the site of a cut. Skin cells wouldn't be able to repair and create new tissue. Traditional medical thinking holds that both this healing process and the energy used in it are beyond our willful control. But what if you could consciously control this supposedly unconscious self-healing process? What if you could learn to harness the most vital component in that process, the healing energy that your body uses to repair itself? What if you could learn to increase and direct that healing energy to improve your general well-being and relieve specific health problems?

This book will give you that ability.

HARNESSING YOUR HEALING ENERGY

Through a series of step-by-step, easy-to-learn, simple-to-perform exercises, you will learn to harness your body's healing energy, the force that is known as *chi* to the Chinese, *mana* to the Polynesians, and *prana* throughout India. You will learn an entire system of self-healing that uses as its framework the principles of one of the most comprehensive, effective forms of energy medicine, called Pranic Healing.

ENERGY MEDICINE

Energy medicine is a broad category of alternative healing methods that utilize universal life force as their primary healing modality. Although some energy medicine is used as an alternative to allopathic, or Western, medicine, most methods are now used as a complement to care given by medical doctors and other traditional treatments. *We strongly recommend that you use Pranic Healing only as an adjunct to your physician's care.*

In energy medicine, good health results from having the right amount of this energy flowing smoothly through the body, while health problems or ailments result from a deficiency or blockage of this energy. Energy medicine typically includes some method of increasing or stimulating the amount of life force in the body to facilitate healing. Some systems advocate drawing in the energy from a source outside the body; others teach practitioners to build up their own vital force and then use that for healing. Some incorporate self-healing; others do not. Acupuncture, *chi kung*, Reiki, Therapeutic Touch, and Pranic Healing are just several examples of energy medicine.

Acupuncture is probably the most well-known energy medicine system today. In acupuncture, fine needles are inserted into a patient's body at certain points, along energy channels called *meridians* (see "Your Energetic Anatomy" below for more on meridians). These needles unblock the flow of life force, or *chi*, through the meridians, and thus balance the body's energy and facilitate healing. Occasionally, the acupuncturist gently rotates the needles or even sends a very low-grade electrical current through them to accelerate the healing process.

Chi kung (literal translation: "energy work") stems from the same Oriental philosophical base as acupuncture, traditional Chinese medicine, and internal Chinese martial arts, such as tai chi. It consists of a variety of life force–generating exercises and practices that date back thousands of years. There are many different types of *chi kung*, but in general, *chi kung* practitioners perform a prescribed set of breathing routines and physical exercises over a period of years to enable them to build up the *chi* in their own bodies. They then project that energy into the body of the patient to bring about healing. You'll learn a different, more effective way to generate energy that is unique to Pranic Healing.

Reiki is a Japanese hands-on energy-channeling system believed to have its origins in the esoteric practices of Tibetan monks. Reiki practitioners must be "attuned" to the universal healing energy by a Reiki master, after which they are able to draw in this life force and allow it to flow through them into the body of a person in need of healing. There are three levels of Reiki training: first degree, second degree, and third degree, or Reiki master.

Therapeutic Touch is a method of energy healing incorporating techniques from traditional Chinese medicine, Ayurveda, and laying on of hands. It was developed in the 1970s by a nurse, Delores Krieger, Ph.D., R.N., at New York University School of Nursing, and Dora Kunz, a healer and author, and is comparable to first-degree Reiki. A Therapeutic Touch practitioner does not actually touch the patient but passes his hands lightly over the patient's body to detect and then "unruffle"—in Therapeutic Touch terminology—energetic blockages. The practitioner then directs energy into the patient to assist healing.

PRANIC HEALING

Pranic Healing was created by a Chinese-Filipino spiritual teacher and energy master named Grandmaster Choa Kok Sui, who spent years researching the root teachings of esoteric systems such as yoga, *chi kung*, Kaballah (an ancient Jewish mystical-spiritual tradition), and many others in order to create a simple, practical, effective, "optimum" energy healing system that anyone could learn and use.

In his teens Grandmaster Choa was already an accomplished student of yoga and various meditation and spiritual systems. In his twenties, he continued intensive study of higher-level esoteric practices, with a particular focus on the use of vital life force for healing. He concluded that healing, at its most basic, consists of cleansing and energizing—that is, cleaning away dirty or blocked life force from the aura and replenishing the aura with fresh energy. Next, Grandmaster Choa, who by this time had also established himself as a businessman and engineer, applied a rigorous scientific approach to his inquiries. He set up a number of healing clinics in the Philippines to test the effectiveness of laying on of hands, *chi kung*, and other energy healing systems. Each patient who came in received a particular type of energetic treatment, and the results—or lack of results—of that particular treatment for that specific ailment were recorded. Grandmaster Choa also had highly skilled healers with heightened sensitivity—people with the ability to see vital life force in the body— observe the patients before and after treatment, so that he could detail the exact energetic effect of each system. These experiments were overseen by nurses and other medical professionals, as well.

These healing clinics continued for years, with Grandmaster Choa constantly testing and refining methods of cleaning out dirty energy and increasing the supply of healing energy. Finally, in 1987, Grandmaster Choa published his first book and held his first workshop in the Philippines to introduce Pranic Healing, a "best of the best" system of very specific instructions and sequences for cleansing and energizing particular parts of the body to achieve rapid healing. The system spread to the United States in 1990 and is now practiced worldwide.

PRANIC HEALING COMPARED WITH OTHER TYPES OF ENERGY MEDICINE

Pranic Healing is a more comprehensive and treatment-specific form of energy medicine than the two more contemporary systems, Reiki and Therapeutic Touch, and it is simpler to learn and easier to apply than the ancient, formal Chinese systems acupuncture and *chi kung*. Additionally, Pranic Healing includes teachings rarely found in other energy medicine systems, such as the detailed use of colored pranas and the practice of *energetic hygiene*.

Like Reiki and Therapeutic Touch, Pranic Healing teaches practitioners to feel for disturbances in the aura. But the Pranic Healing version of this tactile technique, called *scanning*, is more explicit and precise. For instance, Pranic Healing teaches several simple exercises that help students open and sensitize the chakras, or power centers, in the palms of their hands. This enables pranic healers to detect both *congestion*, an energetic blockage, and *depletion*, an energetic deficiency, as they move their hands over the body of a patient. Pranic Healing also includes two other hands-on techniques: *sweeping*, which is manually cleaning away congestion or dirty energy, and *energizing*, which is supplementing areas of pranic insufficiency. Reiki has no comparable sweeping technique, while Therapeutic Touch's unruffling is similar to but not as effective as sweeping. Unruffling resembles what is called in Pranic Healing *distributive sweeping*, or using the hands to move energy gently from one area to another. But Pranic Healing's sweeping provides more focused, complete removal of energetic congestion, primarily because pranic healers can use several types of hand motions in sweeping, depending on the location and "stubbornness" of the energetic blockage.

Energizing is much more detailed in Pranic Healing than in either Reiki or Therapeutic Touch, though it is still simple to learn. Both Reiki and Therapeutic Touch practitioners channel energy into the body of the patient, and there is some rudimentary targeting of the energy to areas where the patient has discomfort, or where the practitioner feels an energetic disturbance. In Pranic Healing, though, for each specific health problem there is a specific sequence for cleaning and energizing particular parts of the body and particular chakras so that the prana is utilized to maximum healing effect.

While it is based upon some of the tenets that underpin both acupuncture and *chi kung*, Pranic Healing is easier to learn and use. As in acupuncture, Pranic Healing works with the meridians, but unlike acupuncture Pranic Healing concentrates on only the largest meridians, along which the major chakras lie. Hundreds of other, smaller meridians crisscross the body, but by performing focused energy work on the large meridians, which feed the others, pranic healers can achieve more effective results in a much shorter period of time. And of course, pranic healers, unlike acupuncturists, needn't study for years to learn the location and path of those smaller meridians and which organs and parts of the body they energize.

There are numerous *chi kung* schools and thus many types of *chi kung* healing techniques. *Chi kung* routines, or "sets" of physical and breathing exercises, were developed by Chinese monks centuries ago to supplement their spiritual development and martial arts training, and also to facilitate physical healing. The biggest differences between *chi kung* and Pranic Healing lie in their energy-generation philosophies and the length of time needed to become proficient in the practice. *Chi kung* relies on internal generation of energy, which means that students learn techniques to help them build up and store energy within their body. They then tap this surplus for meditation, spiritual development, fighting, and healing. Pranic Healing, by contrast, is an external-generation system. Students are taught powerful techniques that enable them to draw in energy from outside the body and then project it into areas of deficiency for healing. Thus, pranic healers don't have to worry about their energy battery "running down." Pranic healers also don't have to spend years learning and practicing complex physical exercises and breathing patterns to build up the level of internal energy needed to heal effectively.

Finally, missing from nearly all other energy medicine systems are two cornerstones of Pranic Healing: the methodical use of colored pranas, which focus and greatly accelerate the healing process, and *energetic hygiene*, or rules and practices for avoiding energetic contamination and keeping the practitioner's personal energy tank clean and full.

YOUR ENERGETIC ANATOMY

Pranic Healing teaches that illness and health problems result from disturbances to the flow of prana through a network of power centers, passageways, and energy fields that interpenetrate the physical body called the *energetic anatomy*. Your energetic anatomy, also called your *energy body*, or simply, your *aura*, is a three-dimensional cloud of prana that begins inside your physical body and emanates outward in all directions to form a rough outline around your body. The energetic anatomy has five basic components:

1. The *chakras*, the body's power centers or transformers that take in and distribute prana.
2. The *meridians*, the body's energy channels that transfer prana to and from the chakras and nearby organs and parts of the body.
3. The *inner aura*, an inner shell of prana that begins inside the body and extends about 5 inches out from the body in a healthy adult.
4. The *outer aura*, an outer shell of prana that also begins inside the body and extends up to several feet beyond the inner aura in a healthy adult. The outer aura holds in the body's energy.
5. The *health aura*, an aggregation of 2-foot-long rays or beams that radiate from the body's pores. In a healthy person, these health rays are straight and well defined, but in a sick person they are crooked or droopy.

These auras are concentric, much like the layers of an onion, with the three auras nesting inside one another (Figure 1–1).

Your energetic anatomy has four principal functions:

1. to absorb, distribute, and energize the physical body with prana;
2. to serve as a mold or template for the physical body;
3. to control, through the chakras, the proper regulation of prana in the physical body;
4. to serve, primarily through the health rays and aura, as a protective shield for the physical body against energetic contamination.

Let's look at the components of the energetic anatomy in more detail.

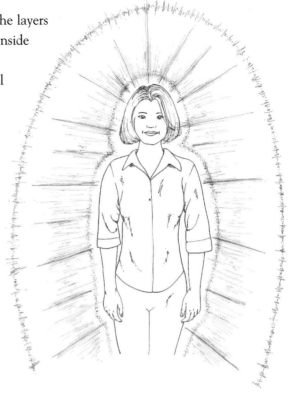

FIGURE 1–1

Chakras

Your energetic anatomy has three types of chakras: major chakras, which are 3 to 4 inches in diameter; minor chakras, which are 1 to 2 inches in diameter; and mini-chakras, which are less than 1 inch in diameter. (*Note:* All sizes are for a healthy adult.)

There are 11 major chakras, three of which—the heart, solar plexus, and spleen—have a front and back aspect. Thus, with the front and back heart, front and back solar plexus, and front and back spleen, you will work with a total of 14 of these major power centers. (You may find it helpful to refer to Figure 1–2a, Figure 1–2b, and Table 1–I as we discuss them.) Starting at the top of the head and working down the front of the body, through the legs and then up the back, the major chakras are: the crown, the forehead, the *ajna* (or brows), the throat, the front heart, the front solar plexus, the front spleen, the navel, the sex, the basic, the *meng mein* (or kidneys), the back spleen, the back solar plexus, and the back heart.

Table 1-I THE ELEVEN MAJOR CHAKRAS			
Chakra	**Location**	**Functions, Corresponding Organs**	**Diseases**
1. CROWN	crown of the head	brain and pineal gland	diseases related to pineal gland and brain, both physical and psychological
2. FOREHEAD	center of the forehead at the hairline	nervous system and pineal gland	loss of memory, paralysis, epilepsy
3. *AJNA*	between the eyebrows	pituitary gland and endocrine glands; controls the other major chakras	cancer, allergy, asthma, and diseases related to the endocrine glands
4. THROAT	center of the throat	throat; thyroid and parathyroid glands	throat-related illnesses such as goiter, sore throat, asthma
5. HEART			
a) front heart	center of the chest at the sternum, or breastbone	heart, thymus gland, and circulatory system	heart and circulatory ailments
b) back heart	on the spine opposite the front heart chakra	lungs and, to a lesser extent, heart	lung problems
6. SOLAR PLEXUS		acts as an energy clearinghouse; also controls the heating and cooling of the body	
a) front solar plexus	solar plexus area, the hollow area just beneath sternum	pancreas, liver, large and small intestines, appendix, stomach	(both front and back solar plexus): high cholesterol, diabetes, ulcer, hepatitis, rheumatoid arthritis, heart ailments, and other illnesses related to these organs
a) back solar plexus	on the spine opposite front solar plexus chakra		

Chakra	Location	Functions, Corresponding Organs	Diseases
7. SPLEEN		spleen	
a) front spleen	left part of the abdomen between front solar plexus chakra and navel; at middle part of left bottom rib	major entry point for air prana; energizes other major chakras and entire body	(both front and back spleen): low vitality, weak body, and blood ailments; autoimmune disorders
b) back spleen	on the back directly opposite the front spleen chakra	same as front spleen	
8. NAVEL	navel	small and large intestines	constipation, difficulty in giving birth, appendicitis, low vitality, and other diseases related to intestines
9. *MENG MEIN*	back of the navel	kidneys, adrenal glands; energizes other internal organs; blood pressure	kidney problems, low vitality, high blood pressure, and back problems
10. SEX	behind the pubic bone	sexual organs, bladder, and legs; lower or physical creative center	sex-related and bladder problems
11. BASIC	base of the spine	Adrenal glands and sex organs; energizes the physical body—bones, muscles, blood, and internal organs; affects general vitality, body heat, and the growth of infants and children; center of self-survival	cancer, leukemia, low vitality, allergy, asthma, sexual ailments, back problems, blood ailments, growth problems

The *minor* and *mini-chakras* are located throughout the body in the jaw, hands, feet, arms, and legs. But since most significant health problems can be addressed by working on the major chakras alone, this book does not discuss in detail the minor and mini-chakras (though several remedies in Chapter 13 refer briefly to them). Here is a brief description of each of the major chakras:

The *crown chakra* is located at the top of the skull and energizes and controls the brain and the pineal gland. It is also one of the most important access points for prana into the body because prana entering the crown energizes the entire body.

The *forehead chakra* is located in the center of the forehead and energizes and controls the nervous system.

The *ajna chakra* is located between the eyebrows and energizes and controls the pituitary gland and endocrine system. The *ajna* is also important because it is the seat of our will power and conscious thought processes.

The *throat chakra* is located at the Adam's apple and controls the throat, trachea, larynx, esophagus, thyroid gland, and lymphatic system. The throat chakra is also connected to the sex chakra, as it is the upper center of creativity, while the sex chakra is the lower center of creativity.

The *heart chakra* is in the center of the chest and has two aspects: a front and a back heart chakra. The front heart chakra is located directly behind the sternum or breastbone. The back heart chakra is located on the spine, between the shoulder blades and directly opposite the front heart chakra. The heart chakra controls the heart, the lungs, and the thymus gland.

The *solar plexus chakra* also has a front and back aspect. The front solar plexus chakra is located in the soft area just below the sternum or breastbone and controls the stomach, pancreas, intestines, and diaphragm. The back solar plexus chakra is located on the spine directly opposite the front solar plexus chakra. The solar plexus chakras are the seat of all our emotions. The front solar plexus controls our expressed emotions—for example, anger that you let out. The back solar plexus controls our suppressed emotions—for example, fears that you bottle up. Because of its connection to the emotions and its proximity to the heart, the front solar plexus chakra also has an energetic and health link to the heart chakra and the physical heart.

The *spleen chakra*, like the heart and solar plexus chakras, has both a front and back aspect. The front spleen chakra is located near the left lowermost rib, or what is called the floating rib. The back spleen chakra is located on the back directly opposite the front spleen chakra. The spleen chakra is important because it draws in prana, assimilates it, and distributes it to all the other chakras.

The *navel chakra* is located at the navel and is one of the body's main power centers. It controls the large and small intestines and affects the birth process. In many Eastern systems, particularly those derived from Taoist teachings, practitioners are taught to focus on the navel chakra during meditation to build up energy.

The *meng mein chakra,* or "gate of life," is located on the back between the kidneys directly opposite the navel chakra. This is a key power center, for it acts as a pumping sta-

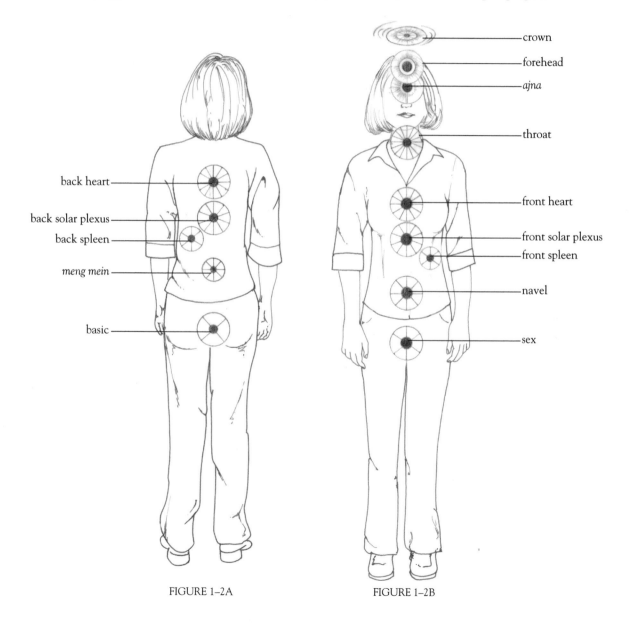

FIGURE 1–2A   FIGURE 1–2B

tion for energy from the basic chakra. It controls the kidneys, adrenal glands, and upper urinary tract, as well as the blood pressure.

The *sex chakra* is located behind the pubic bone. In men, this is behind the base of the penis; in women behind the G-spot. The sex chakra controls the pelvic organs, including the bladder, the prostate (in men), the uterus and ovaries (in women), and the sexual organs.

The *basic chakra* is located at the base of the spine, at the tailbone or coccyx. The basic chakra controls the bones, the muscles, the soft tissue and blood production, as well as the adrenal glands. It also controls the body's general vitality and energy level.

Some forms of yoga, as well as some energy or meditation systems that are concerned primarily with spiritual development, mention only seven chakras. These seven usually include: the root or basic, the spleen, the navel, the heart, the throat, the brow, and the crown. A seven-chakra system may be effective for pure spiritual development, but it is inadequate for physical healing because it omits some important chakras that control and energize key parts of the body—for example, the front and back solar plexus chakras, the sex chakra, and the *meng mein*. Furthermore, it does not acknowledge the front and back aspects of the heart and spleen chakras.

Meridians

Meridians are the body's energy channels. Certain Indian esoteric systems, such as Ayurveda and yoga, refer to these energy channels as *nadis*. Although meridians carry the body's prana, they are not the same as our nervous system, nor do they follow closely the nerve paths or any other physiological paths identified by Western medicine—for example, the circulatory or lymph systems.

The body has several large meridians and hundreds of smaller ones. In this book, we focus on only the two largest channels, for two reasons: first, these two large meridians control the smaller ones; and second, it is along these two major meridians that our major chakras are located. One major meridian runs down the front of the body from the crown on the top of the head down through the heart, front solar plexus, navel, and sex chakras and ends at the perineum (the soft area between the genitals and the anus). In Chinese systems, this meridian is called the *functional channel*. The corresponding major meridian on the back runs up from the perineum through the basic, the *meng mein*, the back solar plexus, the back heart, to the crown. Chinese systems call this the *governor channel*. Those who have read about any Chinese or Taoist systems or practiced them may be familiar with these two channels because together, they comprise what is sometimes called the "microcosmic orbit" or "small heavenly circle." Many Taoist systems feature a meditation that teaches practitioners to circulate their prana through these two large meridians.

Auras

Of your body's three auras—outer, inner, and health—Pranic Healing is most concerned with the inner aura. The inner aura is composed of the prana emanating from the chakras and the meridians. Thus, it is on the inner aura that you perform the energy manipulation techniques of scanning (feeling energetic disturbances), sweeping (cleaning away energetic congestion), and energizing (supplementing areas of pranic deficiency). These techniques are covered in Chapters 5 through 9.

With this discussion of energetic anatomy as a backdrop, let us take a closer look at the bio-force that powers our energetic anatomy, prana.

PRANA

There are three principal sources of prana: the air, from which we get air prana; the earth, from which we get ground prana; and the sun, from which we get solar prana. All living things have the innate ability to absorb and utilize prana to sustain life. We do this unconsciously. For instance, we get solar prana through exposure to sunlight. We get air prana through the act of respiration. And we absorb ground prana through our feet as we walk around every day. (We also get prana from the food we eat, but consuming food is merely an indirect way of obtaining prana that ultimately comes from the air, earth, and sun.)

Other, more powerful, conscious methods of acquiring prana can be employed to obtain both a greater quantity and a higher quality of this life force. These more powerful prana-generation techniques are the key to effective self-healing. Energy generation is discussed in detail in Chapters 8 and 12, but Table 1–II gives you a look at the range of some of these techniques.

While all prana is energy, there are slight variations in the quality of the prana, depending on the source. For instance, solar prana is more refined than ground prana, which means that solar prana vibrates at a higher frequency than earth prana and is composed of smaller, finer particles. While all prana can be used for physical healing, its level of refinement dictates its suitability for certain purposes. For instance, higher-frequency prana

Table 1-II	RANGE OF PRANA-GENERATING TECHNIQUES		
	Low-level Unconscious technique; absorb minimal or sustenance level of prana	**Medium-level** More conscious technique; absorb more prana	**High-level** Focused conscious technique with intent; absorb great quantities of prana
Solar prana	Stand out in sun	Drink clear, clean water that has been left in sun for 24 hours	Open crown chakra through Meditation on Twin Hearts (see Chapter 11) to draw in enormous quantities of solar prana
Air prana	Breathe clean air	Pranic breathing	Water pump technique: Draw prana in through various source chakras using Pranic breathing with proper rhythm and retention; project out through hand; Tibetan Yogic Exercises and Mentalphysics Exercises
Earth prana	Walk around	Walk around barefoot on clean soil	Rooting practices; using chakras on soles of feet to absorb earth prana; Tibetan Yogic Exercises

is used for spiritual development and healing delicate areas, while lower-frequency prana is used for increasing physical power and healing not-so-delicate areas.

Prana is remarkably powerful and resilient, yet it is also very delicate. Prana can be used to relieve serious health problems. It can even be projected over great distances without losing its strength or effectiveness. But your prana can also be diminished or weakened by many factors, including your beliefs, emotions, attitudes, inhibitions, and traumatic memories,

What Physicians Learn in Medical School About Energy

"In four years of medical school, we spent approximately one week in one biochemistry class, during my second year, discussing the body's energy. That week focused narrowly on what is called the Krebs cycle, the molecular process by which cells produce and absorb energy from food.

"We physicians are taught that if a patient comes in complaining of fatigue or low energy, we should run tests to rule out illnesses such as hypothyroidism, diabetes, anemia, and the like. If the tests come back negative and the patient continues to complain, there are two standard diagnoses: depression or stress.

"A diagnosis of depression- or stress-induced fatigue can certainly be true in some cases. And we doctors always want to order the most complete set of tests to rule out serious problems. Even so, the traditional Western medical curriculum does not admit the possibility that there could be a deeper, underlying energetic cause—and cure—for the depression or stress.

"The concepts of complementary and energy medicine are introduced in some medical schools and nursing schools, but medical and nursing curricula still have far too little discussion of the body's overall energy, and virtually no discussion of a healing energy that we can learn to detect, increase, and direct to improve our health—and our patients' health."

—*Eric B. Robins, M.D.*

the food you eat, the people you associate with, where you work and live, *how* you work and live, what you say, what you think, and how you react to the general level of stress in your life.

In general, your state of health is tied to your supply of prana. When your prana is clean and plentiful, you are in good physical and mental health. When your prana is low or dirty, you typically experience some type of health problem.

Now let's perform an experiment that will allow you to feel your own prana.

EXERCISE 1–A: *Detecting Your Own Personal Energetic Anatomy—Hand Sensitivity Exercise 1*

The easiest and quickest way to understand prana and your energetic anatomy, and how simple it can be to work with both, is to learn to *feel* your own personal energy. In this exercise, you will sensitize your hand chakras, which are located in the center of the palm (Figure 1–3), to feel the energy between them. You may sit or stand while performing this exercise.

1. Put your tongue on the roof of your mouth just behind the hard palate (the hard ridge behind your top row of teeth). Keep it there throughout the exercise. This connects the two major energy channels that run down the front and back of your body along which your major chakras are located. It also increases your sensitivity to energy.

2. Take four slow, deep breaths, breathing in and out all the way down to the bottom of your lungs. Breathe in and out through your nose. This helps clear and calm the mind, as well as relax the body.

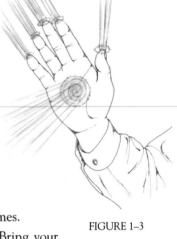

3. *Wrist rolls:* Extend your arms straight out in front of you at shoulder height. Roll your hands at the wrists 10 times in both directions; make small circles with your hands pivoting at the wrist, stirring 10 times clockwise and 10 times counterclockwise.

4. *Hand openers:* Open and close your hands vigorously 10 times.

FIGURE 1–3

5. *Elbow, finger shake:* Begin with your arms at your sides. Bring your fists up near your shoulders as if you were curling a dumbbell in your hands. The back of your hands should be facing away from you. From this position, snap your arms down, flicking your fingers open as you reach the bottom, as if you were dropping the imaginary dumbbells, and then back up 10 times quickly. Take care not to hyperextend your elbow (bend it beyond its natural range of motion) or jolt the joint. This movement should *not* hurt.

6. Extend your hands in front of you, with your palms about 3 inches apart and facing each other as if you are about to clap your hands. Spread your fingers. Now with the thumb of your right hand press down lightly into the center of your left palm for a few seconds. Then repeat the movement with your other hand, using your left thumb to press down into your right palm.

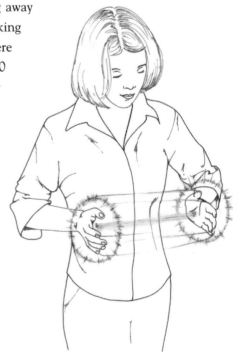

7. Now hold your elbows close to your waist with your forearms extended in front of you, parallel to the ground. Keep your hands relaxed with your palms facing each other about 3 inches apart as if you were

FIGURE 1–4

about to clap your hands. Close your eyes. Keeping your hands a few inches apart, just breathe slowly and focus lightly on the centers of your palms. Do this for about 30 seconds (Figure 1–4).

8. Then, keeping your hands, wrists, and elbows steady, begin to move your arms in and out a few inches from each other, moving your hands closer together and then farther apart. Pretend you are clapping your hands in very slow motion, but don't let your hands meet. Bring your palms to within an inch or two of each other and then, slowly, move them out about a foot, and then bring them close together again. Repeat this action for about 30 seconds. Very shortly, you'll feel some resistance between your palms, as if you're holding a balloon, or your palms will begin to tingle or get itchy or warm. When you do sense this resistance, heat, or buzzing in your hands, what you are feeling is your energy, your prana, the life force that surrounds and interpenetrates the bodies of all living things.

Don't worry if you don't feel this energy on your first try. If you don't sense a warmth or tingling sensation in your palms after completing this exercise once, stop for a few moments, take a few deep breaths, focus on your palms, and start the exercise from the beginning again. You'll feel the energy before too long.

EVEN IF YOU CAN'T FEEL THE ENERGY RIGHT AWAY, RELAX: YOU'LL STILL BE ABLE TO HEAL

We frequently tell our students that those who can't feel the energy immediately can still make this system work for them. Most important, you will still be able to perform healings. When I (Master Co) started with Pranic Healing, I had a technical, skeptical mind (from my engineering training and background), and was hindered further by a strict religious upbringing that did not look favorably upon energy healing. Despite daily practice, I was not able to feel the energy for almost two-and-a-half years. Yet I stayed with the system because I was still able to produce remarkable healings. The incident that really convinced me of the effectiveness of Pranic Healing came when I healed my wife, Daphne, of several compound fractures of her right hip. Daphne had fallen 14 feet, and the orthopedic surgeon who put her in traction to align the bones said it would take at least three-and-a-half months before she could even begin to try to walk again. I began applying Pranic Healing three times daily and subsequent visits to the orthopedic surgeon revealed that her hip was healing rapidly. Finally, in only five weeks—one-third the minimum time her doctor projected—she was up and running, literally. At about the same time, I also relieved my mother's chronic indigestion in only a few minutes, helped several clients reduce lumps by at least 75 percent, and had one client whose liver cancer went into remission for a year. These are dramatic results, but they are just a handful of the healings that I was able to accomplish before I was fully sensitized and able to feel prana. As an instructor over the last ten years, I have witnessed many students who did not immediately feel energy and still were able to relieve their classmates of various aches, pains, and ailments.

The important point to understand is that Pranic Healing is not dependent ultimately on the practitioner's being able to feel energetic disturbances. If you still can't feel prana by the time you get to the specific health remedies in Chapter 13, you can still heal simply by following the step-by-step instructions. Each specific health remedy is a tested, proven "recipe" designed to address the energetic imbalances related to a specific health problem, and you don't need to be able to feel the energy to make the remedy work for you.

As you work through the progressive exercises in this book, if you can't feel the prana, simply relax and continue with the program and your practice. You will feel the energy before too long. The methods of teaching Pranic Healing have improved dramatically over the last ten years. As a result, the vast majority of students today can feel the energy at the end of the first class, and 95 percent can feel their energy within two weeks if they practice hand sensitivity daily. We've based this book on those same new techniques and technologies, so just stick with your practice, and you will feel the prana.

SCIENTIFIC EVIDENCE OF AN ENERGETIC TEMPLATE AND SELF-HEALING ABILITY

While mainstream medicine has been slow—and often outright reluctant—to accept the principles of energy medicine, some medical researchers have conducted experiments that support its basic tenets. Dr. Robert Becker, an orthopedic surgeon at New York University, performed some interesting investigations into the regenerative ability of simple, less evolved life forms that strongly support the notion of an energetic template, or mold. Becker cites the work of Swiss scientist Abraham Trembley, who found several species of hydras (a small, tube-shaped freshwater polyp) that regenerate if cut into pieces, as long as the piece had a portion of the central "stalk" or body. Becker also references at length the experiments of Lazzaro Spallanzani, an Italian priest who showed that a salamander could regrow a tail or a limb if it was cut off. Becker points out that if both the tail and the leg of the salamander are removed, you can take some tail cells and move them to the area of the severed limb, and they will grow into a limb. Before these experiments, it had been thought that these tails cells had differentiated—that is, their genetic code had been programmed to grow into a tail. But the experiments indicate that the salamander's tail cells can de-differentiate (become general cells) and then redifferentiate into cells coded for a different purpose (to grow into a limb). In the salamander body, some force or consciousness in its cells somehow knew to grow a limb, even though the cells that had been placed into the area of the severed limb had already been programmed to grow into a tail. According to traditional scientific thinking, this is not supposed to be possible. Becker compares this to a pile of bricks spontaneously rearranging itself into a high-rise building, complete with structural steel, windows, and roof!

Becker cites further examples of regeneration. A newt can regenerate a new eye, including an optic nerve, in about 40 days. Goldfish and salamanders can regenerate spinal fibers. Even humans have some regenerative capability. The human liver can replace a portion of its mass lost due to injury through what medical science calls compensatory hypertrophy, the ability of cells to increase their rate of division and replace the lost tissue. And damage to or dysfunction of one kidney frequently leads to enlargement of the other.

Becker notes that regeneration becomes more difficult as you move up the evolutionary ladder, but the implications of his work are still significant:

1. Life can heal itself.
2. There is a self-regenerating ability.
3. There is a self-regenerating force and an intelligence that can direct it.
4. There is a larger energetic template that directs cells to grow and differentiate.

BASIC LAWS OF ENERGY SELF-HEALING

Here are the basic principles regarding the use of prana in self-healing. These simple laws underpin the energy and healing work in this book.

1. *When energy flows through the body properly, you are in a state of health.* This is the most fundamental truth about prana, the body, the mind, and our health. If the aura is clean, the meridians clear, and the chakras balanced and functioning properly, the body is in a state of physical and mental health.

2. *When there is an energetic disturbance in the body, a disease state is created.* This is the corollary of the first rule. When the body's energy is disrupted in some way, when it is prevented from flowing smoothly through the meridians, to and from the chakras, and to and from the organs, a health problem is present (or about to be present; see principle 5 below). There are two types of energetic disturbances: congestion, which is an accumulation of either excess or dirty prana; and depletion, which is a deficiency of prana. These energetic disturbances can be either general (occurring throughout the entire aura) or local (occurring in a specific area, chakra or meridian). For the body to be returned to a state of health, these energetic disturbances must be corrected.

3. *You can sense, increase, and direct the body's supply of prana to improve your health—if you have the proper training.* Prana is a living force; it has consciousness. It can be built up and consciously controlled. There is a saying in *chi kung* practice: "The *chi* follows the *yi*." *Chi* is, as explained earlier, a synonym for universal life force. We don't have a perfectly equivalent word for *yi* in English, but it refers to the mind or intent. Thus, the rough translation is: "energy follows thought"; prana goes where you intend it to go. This book provides you with the proper training to build up a surplus of prana and direct it to improve your health.

4. *The body always moves toward homeostasis.* Homeostasis is a word from Greek that means a state of stability or equanimity between different but interdependent groups or elements of an organism. All systems in nature move toward balance. The body, too, seeks a balanced energetic level. Why? Because this state of equilibrium, or health, is our natural state. Our body naturally seeks health.

5. *Illnesses manifest in the energy body before they manifest in the physical body.* The energy body is the template, or mold, for the physical body; it surrounds and interpenetrates the physical body. Thus, health problems occur first as irregularities or disturbances in the energy body before they become symptoms or full-blown health problems in the physical body. By treating problems at the energetic level, you heal the physical body. Additionally, through regular energy-generation exercises and proactive steps to keep the energy body clean, you help prevent physical ailments from occurring and greatly diminish their effects if they do physically manifest.

6. *Healing occurs in the energy body before it becomes apparent in the physical body.* This is a corollary of the fifth principle. When energy healing is applied to the aura, there can often be very rapid and dramatic positive results in the physical body. But there can also be a slight lag time before the healing manifests in the physical body. The length of this lag time depends on factors such as the healer's experience and proficiency, the com-

plexity and severity of the health problem, and the current energy level of the person with the affliction.

7. *The root cause of the energetic disturbances that cause many physical ailments is frequently negative thoughts and emotions stored in the body.* Thoughts, emotions, beliefs, and memories contain real energy that is stored unconsciously in the physical body. (Consider: How do you know when you're nervous, angry, or fearful? Not through intellectual awareness. *Only by feeling a physical manifestation* in your body—for example, stomach spasms, a tight neck, an increased heart rate, a sudden urge to go to the bathroom, heavy perspiration, etc.). Negative emotions themselves do not cause problems; our resistance to feeling them and releasing their energy in a constructive way causes the problem. When you avoid feeling negative emotions and beliefs, your body's musculature physically constricts and holds on to them. Held tightly in the body over a period of time, these negative emotions, limiting beliefs, and traumatic memories form blockages and energetic disturbances that lead to physical health problems. Certainly, your health can be affected adversely by external factors such as bacteria and viruses, as well as poor life choices, bad habits, and accidents. But many health problems result from an energetic disturbance that is ultimately caused by the unconscious mind trapping a negative emotion or limiting belief in the body.

THE SIX STEPS TO SELF-HEALING

This book facilitates self-healing through six steps that help you balance your aura, boost your overall energy, and address particular health problems with specific energetic remedies. As you work through these steps, don't mistake their simplicity for lack of sophistication or effectiveness. Just as the binary system of computer communication, a series of zeroes and ones, appears simple but has enormous brilliance and complexity behind it, these six steps to self-healing are easy to learn and apply because they've been distilled from many powerful energy healing systems and technologies. You're getting only the essential healing practices and techniques, so that you can perform them with minimal preparation and maximum effectiveness. We want you to spend your time healing yourself rapidly and properly, not studying book-length theories. The six steps are:

1. *Clearing negative emotions and limiting beliefs*—This includes several techniques for removing negative emotions, fears, traumatic memories, phobias, anxieties, and limiting

beliefs from the body, where they block the flow of prana. They must be cleared in order to restore the body's energetic balance.

2. *Pranic breathing*—Pranic breathing is an optimal breathing technique that promotes physiological and energetic health benefits, including improved circulation, reduced strain on your heart, an enhanced immune system, and most important, the ability to draw in greater amounts of prana to be used for general energizing and specific self-healing.

3. *Energy manipulation*—These are three unique Pranic Healing techniques. They include *scanning*, the method by which you use your hands to feel for energetic imbalances; *sweeping*, the technique for manually cleaning away dirty or congested prana; and *energizing*, the process of drawing in prana and supplementing depleted areas.

4. *Energetic hygiene*—This is the practice of keeping your energy body as clean and charged up as possible through emotional regulation, dietary recommendations, special physical exercises, breathing practices, meditation, an energetically clean home and work environment, and the appropriate use of salt as a cleansing remedy.

5. *Meditation*—Meditation helps still your mind, calm your body, and increase your flow of healing, cleansing energy. Two meditations are included in this book. One is a mindfulness meditation; the other is Grandmaster Choa's "Meditation on Twin Hearts," a powerful meditation on peace and lovingkindness.

6. *Energy-generation exercises*—These two powerful routines, the modified Tibetan Yogic Exercises and the modified Mentalphysics Exercises, enable you to draw in and generate great quantities of high-quality prana.

In the next chapter, you'll learn about the emotional root cause of many health problems and how your mind's efforts to protect you sometimes aggravate these problems.

CHAPTER 2

The True Nature of Your Mind— How It Protects You and Hurts You

"A thirty-seven-year-old man who'd had chronic prostatitis, an inflammation of the prostate gland, for seventeen years came to see me. His symptoms included urinary frequency and urgency, lower abdominal and testicular pain, and occasional burning during urination, and he was in a great deal of discomfort. Urological studies show that in 92 percent of prostatitis cases, there is no associated infection—that is, the prostate is inflamed, but tests don't reveal any medical problem. We physicians call this kind of problem a 'functional disorder.'

"I told this man that we frequently store negative emotions in the body, and that they can cause actual physical problems, including functional disorders, such as prostatitis. In the course of our conversation, he said that his mother was very abusive toward him when he was growing up, and that he had a tremendous amount of anger about it, but he had 'held it in' for years.

"I explained that his resisting feeling those negative emotions over the years had likely contributed to weaknesses in his health. We worked together for one session, using direct clearing methods to address his pent-up anger. Shortly thereafter, he was symptom-free for the first time in nearly two decades. At subsequent follow-ups, he remained symptom-free."

—ERIC B. ROBINS, M.D.

In a typical visit to a doctor, a patient might complain of a headache, insomnia, backache, vague stomach or abdominal discomfort, or urinary problem. The physician, being a scientist and wanting to be thorough, notes the patient's symptoms and conducts an examination. He or she then offers what is called the "differential diagnosis," which is the spectrum of possible reasons for the symptoms, ranging from the simplest and least problematic to the most severe and life-threatening. The doctor bases the differential diagnosis on his experience observing these symptoms, their frequency, location, and severity, as well as the patient's medical history. For example, the differential diagnosis for a headache might include sinus headache, muscle tension caused by poor posture at a person's desk, migraine, and even a brain tumor. One differential diagnosis for abdominal discomfort might include indigestion, mild food poisoning, irritable bowel syndrome, an ulcer, or the early stages of stomach cancer.

The doctor then orders a few diagnostic tests to check for any serious illnesses.

Several days later, the doctor calls the patient with the results, and the news is good. "All your tests are negative; there's nothing wrong," the doctor says. The patient is relieved that there is no serious problem but then asks, "Why am I still having symptoms if 'nothing's wrong'?"

The doctor replies, "Well, we're really not sure," and again tries to reassure the patient that this condition, though without an apparent cause, is nothing serious. The doctor continues, "If your symptoms are creating too much discomfort, we can give you something to help you feel better." This usually means a prescription—for example, extra-strength Motrin for severe headaches, muscle relaxers for back or neck tension, or a stomach acid inhibitor such as Tagamet for indigestion, to name a few popularly dispensed medications. These remedies may or may not relieve the symptoms.

Thus, the patient often comes away from the encounter without any real understanding of the problem, its cause, or what can be done about it, other than to take medicine to control the symptoms.

Seventy percent of all visits to a primary care physician proceed like this, with patients seeking treatment for difficult-to-diagnose problems called *functional disorders*, which are ailments that cause real, discernible symptoms but that present no medically detectable cause: no virus, bacteria, tumor, mass, or structural abnormality. Functional disorders include problems such as irritable bowel syndrome and many other types of gastrointestinal complaints, many types of headaches and backaches, many types of urinary urgency and frequency, many types of pelvic pain in women, and so on. These problems are termed "functional" because, despite a lack of perceptible pathology, the body's functioning is disrupted. Even though there is no apparent reason for the symptoms, however, people with functional disorders still suffer real pain and discomfort. Crushing headaches can prevent them from leading a normal life; chronic gastrointestinal upsets can interfere with their ability to enjoy many foods; painful back spasms can render them bedridden; the overpowering and sometimes embarrassing need to go to the bathroom may occur at inconvenient or difficult times.

Even though they willingly prescribe medications to control these symptoms, many physicians believe that people with functional disorders either are exaggerating their complaints (hypochondria) or are stressed out, depressed, or anxiety-ridden. In other words, these physicians believe that such ailments are "all in the patient's head."

Functional disorders and many health problems *are* in our head because our "head"—or more properly, our mind—is actually located throughout our entire body. Our mind is inseparable from our body, so if we have a health problem in our head/mind, we've also got one in our body. This is the essence of the *mind-body connection*, which refers to a different, deeper understanding of a disorder that's "in a patient's head."

THE MIND-BODY CONNECTION

There is certainly ample proof that we accept intuitively the link between mind and body. For example, we say, "you'll worry yourself sick," and "I was so stressed out I couldn't sleep," both of which demonstrate a belief that the mind can produce a physical effect on the body. Even the physician who orders up a drug that he knows will only relieve the symptoms of an ailment he believes is caused by stress is acknowledging that this person somehow is thinking himself sick.

Medical research is turning up harder scientific evidence that this mind-body link is not only intuitive, it's physiological. The most compelling data may come from Dr. Candace Pert, a psychoneuroimmunologist who has studied the effect of the mind and emotions on health. Dr. Pert's work has focused on biochemicals called "neuropeptides," which were found to be "messenger molecules" that carry the signals or commands from the brain to every cell in the body. Dr. Pert discovered that these neuropeptides act like keys that fit into locks, or specific sites on cells, called receptors. These receptors were found to cover the surface of all the cells in the body, including the immune system, the endocrine system, and those parts of the body controlled by the autonomic nervous system (ANS). The ANS regulates many of the functions in our bodies that happen involuntarily, such as pulse rate, breathing, sweating, digestion, and blood flow, among others. Neuropeptides help us run our automatic bodily processes. They carry messages that tell the cells in the lungs to breathe in and out, the cells in the adrenal glands to release adrenaline, and so on.

These neuropeptides also carry, according to Dr. Pert's research, commands for our emotions. Thus, if someone is happy or sad or angry, a certain neuropeptide would carry that particular feeling throughout the body. While the definitive experiment that would identify in a rigorously scientific way which neuropeptide carries which emotion has yet to be devised, Dr. Pert nonetheless feels confident enough to assert that these neuropeptides are the "biochemical correlates of emotion." Dr. Pert also states that this system of messenger molecules and receptors represents a "psychosomatic communication network" that is the physiological link between the mind, the emotions, and the body. Messenger molecules are basically "chakra juice," she says. "The chemicals that mediate emotion and the receptors for those chemicals are found in every cell in the body."

Thus, modern medicine demonstrates scientifically what we know intuitively: that the mind is located throughout the body.

THE UNCONSCIOUS MIND

But we don't have just one mind located throughout the body. We actually have two minds, or if you prefer, two parts to one mind: the *conscious mind* and the *unconscious mind*, which is the mind that is our primary focus for health.

The conscious mind is our will, our here-and-now awareness. It is the part of the mind we use to set goals and perform rational evaluations. When you are instructed later on in the book to "use your intent" at the outset of various exercises, it is your conscious mind you will use.

The unconscious mind is that part of our mind that remains outside our conscious awareness. It carries out its mental duties without volition or will on our part. Here are the unconscious mind's primary responsibilities: First, it regulates all of our nonconscious bodily functions. The unconscious mind automatically controls our heartbeat, blood flow, breathing, brain function, endocrinological secretions, and all other organic operations of our body that would be impossible to control with conscious effort. Second, the unconscious mind stores our emotions, memories, behaviors, and knowledge, both individual and collective. These mental archives include our personal history, which consists of all our learnings, experiences, and influences—good and bad, positive and negative, whether they took place repeatedly over a lifetime or for a few fleeting but perhaps traumatic seconds. They also include our collective history, which consists of the memories, behaviors, and learnings we share as members of the human race. Some schools of psychology call this our "collective unconscious." Third, the unconscious mind controls the flow of prana throughout the body. It absorbs, assimilates, and distributes prana throughout the energy body that surrounds and interpenetrates the physical body. Fourth, and perhaps most important to our discussion of health and illness, the unconscious mind strives to protect us from harm, danger, and pain.

How the Unconscious Mind "Protects" Us

The human species has evolved over hundreds of thousands of years, and we retain certain vestiges of our prehistoric ancestors' makeup. Some of these remnants are physical—for instance, the appendix serves no biological purpose today, but nonetheless we still have it. Many more of these remnants, however, are mental or emotional directives that have been hardwired into our unconscious mind. Foremost among these is its primary directive: to protect us and ensure our survival. This instinct is a mental relic from prehistoric times when our ancestors had to fight every day to survive. This protection/survival impulse is evident in our innate drive to procreate and our will to live. It also manifests as responses that help ensure our emotional or psychological survival, in coping mechanisms that help us "survive" negative emotions, traumatic memories, and harmful or limiting beliefs.

Ironically, though, the unconscious mind's principal emotional or psychological survival strategy can be a significant *cause* of health problems: It suppresses the hurtful thought, belief, feeling, or emotion from coming to conscious awareness, so that we won't have to reexperience the pain we originally felt. To offer a common example, nearly everyone grows up getting the clear message that it's not okay to feel or express certain emotions, such as anger. If you cry out of anger or frustration as a child, an impatient parent may yell at you to "shut up!"; a teacher may make you stand in the corner; or your classmates may tease you. As these incidents are repeated over time, we learn—our unconscious mind is programmed—to suppress our anger because we don't like to be yelled at, punished, or ridiculed; these things cause us pain. The unconscious mind also often buries our traumatic memory of the original incidents that led to the programming—in this case, with parents, teachers, and classmates—because these recollections, too, would cause us pain.

The unconscious mind means well in "protecting" us from this pain, but this suppression creates what neural physicist and researcher Dr. Paul Goodwin has called a "functional boundary," which occurs when some *emotional* disturbance, strongly held or suppressed in the musculature of the body, creates an *energetic* disturbance that inhibits the smooth flow of prana. Without an adequate supply of energy, the part of the body with the functional boundary *malfunctions*—it experiences either energetic congestion or depletion—and illness or a health problem can arise.

The three most common unconscious emotional survival strategies are: resisting feeling negative emotions, "clamping down," and forming limiting beliefs.

Resisting Feeling Negative Emotions

Noted psychologist Gay Hendricks, Ph.D., believes that "all negative emotions are gentle, short-lived waves." Yet many people can attest to the intensity and longevity of their fears: worries about job uncertainties or money; anger felt since childhood at parents or siblings; insecurities about personal appearance; the throat-tightening phobia about public speaking. How can they all be nothing more than mild blips of mental energy that come and go quickly? These are the kinds of negative emotions that tie people into knots trying to cope with them.

But there's a second part to Hendricks' definition: "All negative emotions are gentle, short-lived waves, *unless we resist feeling them*." It is our inability to acknowledge and feel negative emotions in our body—not the negative emotion itself—that creates functional boundaries to the smooth flow of prana.

Resisting negative emotions is also called denial. Let's talk about how we handle fear. In our society, it's unacceptable for anyone to feel and express fear, especially men. This is universal cultural programming. That doesn't stop us from *being* afraid of heights, spiders, public speaking, death, losing our job, or any one of hundreds of possible fear or phobia triggers. After all, it is quite human to be afraid. However, we are frequently disdainful of anyone who admits to fear, which is identified with being soft, weak, or overly sensitive. So, in a society in which we mustn't show fear, we learn (and in learning, we are programmed) at virtually every turn—from parents, schoolteachers, coaches, peers, and other authority figures—not to feel and express fear in *any* way. Our unconscious mind's survival instinct kicks in to "protect" us from feeling all fear, and thus buries any fears or phobias that we may have deep in our body, far from conscious awareness. Once buried and suppressed, these fears and phobias can create functional boundaries, which inhibit the flow of prana and can lead to health problems.

We do feel the *effects* of fear in our body, such as the racing heart, dry mouth, and tight stomach when we feel afraid, but only after the negative emotion has built to such an intensity that it bursts through our unconscious defenses. By the time we feel the physical effects of a negative emotion in our body, that means the emotion has overridden our unconscious survival mechanism and has created an energetic disturbance. At this point, a physical health problem may be imminent.

"Clamping Down"

If you experienced a traumatic event when you were young—for example, you were physically abused or grew up in a war-torn country—those memories are stored in your unconscious mind and, thus, throughout your entire body. In order to prevent these memories from surfacing to your conscious mind, where they would be replayed, your unconscious mind, acting on its prime directive to protect us, frequently "clamps down" on the memory: it contracts or constricts tightly the smooth muscles or internal organ where the memory is stored. Clamping down is a specific type of resistance to feeling negative emotions. Here are some examples of how clamping down creates functional boundaries that prevent the proper flow of prana and can ultimately lead to health problems:

- If your unconscious mind clamps down on the smooth muscles of the air passages of the lungs, this can become asthma.
- If your unconscious mind clamps down on the smooth muscles of the bladder, this can become urinary urgency or frequency.
- If your unconscious mind clamps down on the smooth muscles of the blood vessels, this can become high blood pressure. If it clamps down on specific blood vessels to the brain, this can lead to a migraine headache.
- If your unconscious mind clamps down on the smooth muscles of the intestinal tract, this can become irritable bowel syndrome, producing vague abdominal pain, bloating, diarrhea, or constipation.

(Note that all these ailments are functional disorders. This is why functional disorders are so tough to detect through most medical tests. Their origin is emotional and energetic rather than anatomic.)

The unconscious mind doesn't clamp down only on smooth muscles over which we have no conscious control, however. It can also clamp down and create functional boundaries in striated muscle—the larger structural muscles over which we do have voluntary control, as the work of Dr. John Sarno, a professor of physical medicine at New York University, has demonstrated.

In his practice, Dr. Sarno sees patients with the world's worst chronic pain: people who have had debilitating pain in their neck, shoulder, back, or legs for 20 or 30 years; people who have had multiple surgeries and multiple attempts at epidural pain relief (injections into the spine). Frequently they have had an MRI scan that reveals a serious anatomic abnormality such as a slipped disc, spinal arthritis, or spinal cord stenosis (narrowing of the channel through which the spinal cord passes). Nearly all of his patients have been told by another doctor that it is this anatomic abnormality that is causing their pain.

Yet with this group of 20,000 patients, some of whom he has been following for up to 25 years, he has a remarkable 88 percent cure rate. An additional 10 percent of his patients are classified as much improved. He has achieved these remarkable results without surgery or any traditional medical remedy. Instead, he bases his treatment plan on two radical premises: first, he rejects the traditional medical cause-and-effect relationship between anatomical defects and pain; and second, he treats the pain as emotionally based tension caused by striated muscles clamping down, a problem he calls "Tension Myofascial Syndrome," or TMS.

Sarno exhaustively reviewed the medical literature on chronic pain and found numerous studies showing that if you perform an MRI scan on 100 middle-aged people with no back pain, you'll find that 40 to 50 percent of them have a slipped disk just as a matter of course. Additionally, he found studies revealing that people who *did* have abnormal MRI scans, which showed significant anatomic abnormalities, such as slipped disks, spinal arthritis, or stenosis, were no more likely to develop musculoskeletal pain in the future than people whose MRI scans were normal.

From these studies, he developed his theory: The proximate cause of structural pain is muscles clamping down on nerves and limiting the blood flow into the afflicted area, which leads to local hypoxia, or lack of oxygen. But the ultimate cause is the person's inability to regulate and reconcile negative emotions, principally anger, because it's these negative emotions held tightly in the body that are causing the muscles to clamp down.

Sarno asserts that it is a generally accepted societal norm that it is not okay for people to feel their negative emotions, especially anger. When anger wells up, as it does for everyone from time to time, the unconscious mind, in its sincere but misguided attempt to protect us and help us survive in a world in which such emotions are not appropriate, says, "It's not okay to be feeling this anger." The unconscious mind then "protects" us by causing certain muscles to clamp down and generate pain in order to divert attention away from our anger.

Sarno's treatment consists of having his patients come to two lectures. His principal messages are that it's *not* a slipped disk or bone spur that is causing the pain, and that a different view of how to remedy the pain is required for healing. Sarno instructs his patients to stop babying their back and taking pills when they feel pain. Instead, they should ask themselves what they're angry about. Additionally, and perhaps most important, Sarno also tells them that they don't have to get rid of their anger in order to be free of the pain, just their resistance to *feeling* the anger.

Limiting Beliefs

If, as a child, you saw that your parents weren't really happy in their lives, and there was a great deal of fighting and yelling at home all the time, what type of beliefs do you think you might form about marriage?

If, when you were a little girl, you had your heart set on being a dancer, yet you weren't terribly coordinated and the instructor told you "really don't have a dancer's body," what beliefs do you think you might develop about your own sense of self?

If you consistently brought home report cards with six As and one B, yet your father repeatedly berated you for not having all As, how do you think you'd feel about any future efforts that weren't perfect?

All these are examples of ways we develop limiting beliefs.

Limiting beliefs are mental judgments that we've made about ourselves, the way the world works, or the way we interact in the world based on faulty, incomplete, or improperly understood information we have received, typically in the formative years of childhood. This information can come from primary authority figures (parents, teachers, clergy) or peers (classmates, friends), or indirectly from other sources in the world (books, television, movies, advertising). This information may be true on some level. Perhaps your parents' marriage wasn't very good and loving, or you really didn't have the ability to be a dancer. The information may even be well-intended. Your father may have honestly believed he was trying to motivate you to settle for nothing less than your best effort. The mind of a child lacks the ability to discriminate and sort through these messages, however, so these unfiltered messages impinge upon your unconscious mind and lead you to form untrue assumptions about yourself and the world. These gross generalizations become *limiting beliefs*, which, in some ways, are the toughest types of unconscious programming to dislodge or bypass.

The primary way in which limiting beliefs create health problems for you is through the negative emotions, stress, and frustration they produce when you try to act against them in the course of living your life. Using the examples above, here is how limiting beliefs create negative emotions that lead to health problems:

- If, as a result of a less-than-satisfying home life when you were growing up, you formed the limiting belief that "no one can be happy in marriage," you may well have continuing relationship problems throughout your adult life. You may end up with someone with whom you're incompatible. Or you may have a series of unhappy relationships or marriages. You may grow angry, bitter, and resentful, unable to give or accept love.

- If, because you were unable to become a successful dancer, you formed the limiting belief that that you were "no good at anything," you may filter many of your life choices through that belief. You may end up under-achieving in many areas, settling for jobs, relationships, and situations that you know aren't the best for you. You may develop chronic self-doubt and become frustrated at every turn, lacking the confidence to strive for what you really want and without the ability to be happy with what you have achieved.

- If your father's haranguing you about your good-but-not-perfect report card caused you to form the belief that "I have to be perfect in everything I do," you may go through life with unrealistic expectations, always counting on yourself and everyone around you to be flawless. In an imperfect world with imperfect people and imperfect efforts, that's a formula for a life of disappointment, anger, and unhappiness.

THE UNCONSCIOUS MIND IS NEUTRAL, BUT YOU CAN "GET IT ON YOUR SIDE"

The unconscious mind is neutral. It is neither "on your side" nor "against you." It is often said that the unconscious mind functions much like a computer, carrying out its duties in accordance with the information that is loaded into it. Most of its programs are beneficial, or at least have a positive or utilitarian aspect. For instance, it's a good thing that you don't have to think consciously to control your respiration. Some of its programs have both positive and negative implications. For example, it's also good that, when we are in a life-threatening situation, we don't have to activate with conscious thought all the bodily changes that we need to occur to save ourselves. But, as you read earlier, this protection impulse of the unconscious mind can go too far and cause problems. Finally, each of us has many other programs, as well, that we have learned, developed, or had imprinted upon us in the course of living our lives and coming under the influence of parents, schools, peers, the media, and other authority figures. They're unique to us. Some of these deeply hidden programs, as you saw in this chapter, can be the root cause of many physical and emotional ailments.

But here's the good news: You can reprogram the unconscious mind. Even though your unconscious mind may have created programs that cause you personal conflicts, relationship difficulties, or health problems, these programs *can* be altered or bypassed; you can get your unconscious "back on your side." You can clear out the negative emotions, traumatic memories, and limiting beliefs that are evidence of harmful programming—and that cause many health problems—by learning to communicate with your unconscious in the right way. You'll learn two such powerful communication techniques in Chapter 3.

SUMMARY OF ENERGETIC AND EMOTIONAL CAUSES OF HEALTH PROBLEMS

Here is a summary of the key points in Chapters 1 and 2 regarding the energetic and emotional causes of health problems:

1. We have an energetic anatomy, or energy body, that surrounds and interpenetrates the physical body. This energy body also acts as a mold or template for the physical body.
2. The unconscious mind is the central repository of our thoughts, feelings, beliefs, emotions, and memories—both positive and negative.
3. The unconscious mind is located throughout the entire physical body via a neurobiochemical messengering system. At this physiological level, the unconscious mind delivers commands to the parts of the body concerned with our involuntary functions; it also carries our thoughts, feelings, beliefs, emotions, and memories to all parts of the body.
4. The unconscious mind is also located throughout the entire physical body via the energy body. At this energetic level, the unconscious mind regulates and controls the flow of prana through the body.
5. We have an unconscious mind that behaves somewhat like a "neutral computer." It acts according to the data, or programming, that has been entered into it. We have programs hardwired into our unconscious mind, and we have programs that we have learned or picked up in the course of living our lives. These programs may or may not be beneficial for us, but negative or harmful programs can be altered or bypassed. The unconscious mind can be reprogrammed by learning how to communicate with it properly.
6. The unconscious mind can and does place in the physical body negative emotions such as fear or anger, memories of personal traumas, limiting beliefs about our insecurities and personal sense of self-worth, and the everyday worries and anxieties of life and work. It doesn't do this maliciously, but rather, out of a desire to "protect" us from having the

pain of these emotions and events brought back to conscious awareness, where we'd have to relive them.

7. Resisting feeling these negative emotions, traumatic memories, and limiting beliefs can create energetic disturbances called functional boundaries, which are barriers to the smooth flow of prana necessary for good health. These energetic disturbances act like boulders in a creek. Upstream, there is a backup and overflow; downstream, the flow is reduced to a trickle. In your energetic anatomy, these disturbances correspond to energetic congestion and depletion.

8. The physical body responds to the energetic disturbance with more muscular tension, resistance, and strain, which feed the cycle of resistance and energetic disturbance.

9. The intensity of the energetic disturbance—either congestion or depletion or a combination of both—increases until, finally, a physical health problem arises.

In the next chapter, you'll learn the first of the six healing steps, *clearing negative emotions and limiting beliefs*, a range of techniques specifically designed to address the energetic, unconscious, and emotional origins of health problems.

Part II

The Six Steps to Self-Healing

Step 1: Clearing Negative Emotions and Limiting Beliefs (Chapter 3)

Step 2: Pranic Breathing (Chapter 4)

Step 3: Energy Manipulation (Chapters 5 through 9)

Step 4: Energetic Hygiene (Chapter 10)

Step 5: Meditation (Chapter 11)

Step 6: Energy-Generation Exercises (Chapter 12)

CHAPTER 3

All Clear!—
Removing
Emotionally Based
Energetic Blockages

"The chart of one of my patients showed that she sought help for numerous problems, including constipation, insomnia, asthma, migraine headaches, and high blood pressure. All these problems involved tension in the smooth muscles of her body: gastrointestinal tract, lungs, and blood vessels. As we spoke, it was obvious that she had a lot of stress in her life. She had to take care of her aged and ill mother—cooking, feeding, bathing, and medicating her. She also had a husband who was overly dependent and demanding. When I asked this patient how she felt about all of these drains on her time and energy, she replied wearily, 'I don't know.' She told me that she'd decided consciously, as a young child, to repress and not feel such emotions, and certainly not to reveal to others how she was feeling. She told me that her husband had no idea about everything she did for her mother; nor was he aware of her resentment of his demanding ways. When I worked with her to help her become aware of her feelings, suggesting that it was okay for her to feel the truth of what she was feeling in her body, she seemed astonished. But then, in the next moment, she accepted this suggestion. In that split-second, her self-awareness of how her mind actually worked and her positive acceptance of her negative emotions caused a tremendous physiological shift in her body. She told me later that, at an appointment that same day with her internist, her blood pressure measured 146/78. In her entire adult life her blood pressure had never dropped below 170/95. It was her self-awareness of her negative emotions that enabled her to make this physiological shift and bring about a significant reduction in her blood pressure."

—ERIC B. ROBINS, M.D.

I f you've ever attempted to use your conscious mind to overcome fears, anxieties, or limiting beliefs, you likely tried one of three remedies: *denying*, or suppressing them from conscious awareness; *diverting*, or replacing the negative thought with positive thoughts; or *distracting*, engaging in compulsive activity so that you won't notice them. And if you did try one of these three popular remedies, you also likely found out that it helped you feel better for a while, but did not permanently remove the negative emotion or belief. As you read in Chapter 2, denying or suppressing a negative emotion only gives it more power because your unconscious mind buries the feelings even deeper. Diverting your attention through repetition of positive affirmations may enable you to overcome mild fears temporarily. For deep-seated anxieties and rooted beliefs, though, it's like applying a fresh coat of paint over an old surface without scraping and priming first; it won't last. Distracting yourself by taking drugs, drinking, gambling, having excessive sex, becoming a workaholic, or immersing yourself in a hobby is nothing more than avoidance. The problem doesn't go away; you're just hiding from it. Denying, diverting, and distracting don't provide lasting results because they are attempts at conscious denial of an unconscious problem. If you try consciously to disavow or block off your unconscious emotions and beliefs, you're fighting yourself. This only increases the resistance.

If you learn to communicate properly with your unconscious mind, which means acknowledging, accepting, and feeling your negative emotions, limiting beliefs, and traumas, you can permanently rid yourself of them—you can alter or bypass negative programming—and the mental anguish and physical health problems they cause. This is the first of the six steps to self-healing: *clearing negative emotions and limiting beliefs*.

DIRECT AND INDIRECT CLEARING

There are two basic clearing methods: *direct* and *indirect*. A *direct* method is designed specifically to clear emotional and energetic blockages. An *indirect* method provides a variety of energetic or healthful benefits, one of which is clearing negative emotions.

Direct methods include the two simple exercises in this chapter: *self-awareness*, a cognitive technique that helps you constructively acknowledge and feel emotional disturbances; and *higher-level thinking*, a rapid method of getting an objective perspective on negative behaviors and habits. As first explained by Gay Hendricks, Ph.D., in his book, *At the Speed of Life: A New Approach to Personal Change Through Body-Centered Therapy*, direct clearing methods work primarily by having you place nonjudgmental awareness on a problem for a period of time. Putting neutral attention on the thought or emotion removes its power; the blockage is "starved" of energy, it eventually dissolves, and your negative programming is effectively neutralized or bypassed.

Indirect methods include pranic breathing (Chapter 4), the energy manipulation techniques of scanning, sweeping, and energizing (Chapters 5 through 9), energetic hygiene (Chapter 10), and meditation (Chapter 11). Each of these indirect methods clears negative emotions in a slightly different way, as you will see in the cited chapters.

Both direct and indirect methods are effective in clearing negative emotions and limiting beliefs, though they differ in how clearing is achieved. Clearing with a direct method is usually more dramatic and sudden; indirect methods are usually more subtle and gradual. These aren't hard-and-fast rules, however. For example, pranic breathing is a relatively passive, simple technique that produces incremental positive changes in your energy and health, but it can produce powerful results. Many people experience abrupt, rapid emotional clearing through changing their breathing patterns alone. Another example: Self-awareness can bring about sudden insights into your emotions, motivations, and behaviors, leading to startlingly quick clearing of complexes. Self-awareness can also work at a more moderate rate, however, promoting positive changes in behavior, energy, and health over a longer period of time. Or it can work so gradually that one day you simply become aware that some situation or stimulus that used to bother you no longer does.

None of this means that direct methods are any more or less effective than indirect methods. It simply means that clearing takes place in different ways and at different paces for each person. The speed of clearing depends on the complexity of the health problem, how long you've had it, how deeply seated the root disturbance is, your aptitude for the techniques, and how frequently and how well you apply them.

YOUR GOAL: INTEGRATION

Your goal in clearing work, whether you use a direct or an indirect method, is to achieve true, long-lasting positive changes so that you no longer feel the physical symptoms in your body. This is a state of full *integration*, a state of health in which negative emotions and limiting beliefs, as well as the energetic blockages they've created, are gone. Your mind and body are working together, you've overcome any negative programs you've acquired, and prana is flowing smoothly and abundantly.

True integration occurs only at the level of the unconscious mind because, as noted earlier, this is where negative emotions and limiting beliefs reside. It's difficult, however, for us to get in close touch with our unconscious mind to clear these disruptions. Clearing and integration require *conscious-unconscious dissociation*, or separation between your conscious mind (and its willfulness and rational thought), and your unconscious mind (and its emotions, beliefs, and memories). Dissociation gives us perspective on the workings of the unconscious mind. Here's an example of perspective: Have you noticed how easy it is to give advice to a friend or acquaintance, even on a particularly difficult or challenging problem? He may be faced with a really tough decision: whether to change jobs, whether to get a divorce, what to do with a child who's having problems at school. Yet most of us can coolly analyze the situation and often quickly offer a solution. If it were *our* problem, though, if we were facing the same circumstances, we might spend inordinate amounts of time analyzing the problem, considering and reconsidering the options, researching the details, and seeking out the opinions of family, friends, counselors, and perhaps even professionals. And even after conducting research and soliciting opinions, we still might procrastinate, delay, or even avoid making the tough decision. Why? Because we're too close to it, too vested in the outcome to be objective. We're thinking about the consequences that will follow no matter which course we choose. But when the choice belongs to someone else and we don't have a full stake in the result, it's easier to distance ourselves from the end result and make a decision much more quickly.

That's the objectivity you need to remove negative emotions and limiting beliefs. Proper awareness is the key to getting that objectivity.

Awareness

In the West, we tend to relate awareness to one of the five senses. But the awareness you need to develop to clear negative emotions doesn't involve the ability to see or hear things; rather, it is more akin to what Zen literature calls *mindfulness*: a sustained, watchful state of sensitivity, in which you're open and receptive to sensations that arise within.

Awareness can be achieved only through *letting go* of conscious thought and active sensing. Otherwise, the conscious mind overrides the unconscious mind and suppresses this heightened inner sense. Awareness is similar to self-hypnosis, which is really just a state in which you improve your rapport with your unconscious mind. For example, when people perform self-hypnosis, they allow the mind and the body to relax, and they get more in touch with impulses from their unconscious minds. Awareness is also nonjudgmental, which means that as you turn your awareness upon a negative emotion or belief, you hold no thoughts of blame toward yourself or anyone else, nor do you ascribe to it a good or bad quality. For instance, if you are using self-awareness to clear a compulsive need to be perfect, which often causes people to be hypercritical of others and themselves, you might suddenly reexperience the pain of being harshly criticized by your parents for minor transgressions, or the overwhelming feeling of failure you felt when you were cut from junior high cheerleader tryouts. As these emotions resurface—and they will, for if they don't, you can't clear them—you simply note them *without reacting to them*. This means that as these experiences come up, you don't blame your parents for being critical, and you don't wallow in the embarrassment you felt at the age of thirteen. You train yourself just to be aware of them.

Awareness is difficult for Westerners to accept because we're a society that values aggressiveness and action. We have a don't-just-sit-there-do-something approach to problem-solving. We scoff at the apparent passivity of mindfulness and awareness, which can seem to represent a don't-just-do-something-sit-there attitude. As you practice awareness in these direct clearing techniques, however, you will come to realize its powerful healing capability.

TWO DIRECT CLEARING TECHNIQUES

Direct clearing techniques are simply a way to communicate formally with your unconscious mind or inner self. The key to effective communication is understanding that the communication may or may not be verbal. Your "inner critic," that harsh little voice in your mind that blames you for making a minor mistake, usually communicates in words. But other parts of your inner self may "speak" to you through pictures or images. You may also get an impression, feeling, or physical twinge as you practice the direct clearing techniques. Here are several examples of how various feelings might manifest to you, using the example of the excessive need for perfectionism cited above. As you turn your self-awareness on the problem, you might hear your father's voice as he criticized you for your shortcomings—in the exact tone and words he used. Or, you might feel your stomach tightening up as the anger and fear you felt back then resurface. Perhaps you'd see a picture of yourself as a little girl walking home from school dejectedly the day you didn't make the cheerleading squad, and you feel your shoulders actually slump as you reexperience those feelings of failure. Or, you might hear a little voice—perhaps your father, the cheerleading coach, or even yourself—telling you, "You're no good."

Self-Awareness

When practicing awareness, you lightly place your attention on the feelings in your body that a particular emotion, belief, thought, or trauma generates. Awareness is the opposite of resistance. You don't fight the emotion. You don't try to convince yourself it's not there. You acknowledge and feel it in an objective, constructive way. For example, if your inner critic—in your own voice or in the voice of some other authority figure—begins to berate you, and you feel your stomach tighten in response, you simply lightly place your awareness on that feeling. You don't consciously "debate" the voice, and you don't divert or distract your attention away from the discomfort in your stomach in an effort to relieve it. Nor do you consciously try to relax your stomach. You simply be with the tightness, and note that it is there, and that you are aware of it. In essence, you are saying, "This feeling in my stomach is neither good nor bad. It's just the way things are at this particular moment." And then you stay with the feeling as long as you can. Above all else, awareness is nonjudgmental.

Feeling negative emotions doesn't mean getting weepy every time you encounter a situation that makes you afraid. Nor is it wallowing in the emotion so intensely that you're paralyzed by its intensity or driven into despair, depression, or self-pity. You simply give yourself permission to feel your feelings and the sensations they cause in your body without judgment or blame.

A Few Notes on Practicing the Self-Awareness and Higher-Level Thinking Exercises That Follow.

- The right length of time for these sessions is 15 to 20 minutes. A session longer than that may make you tired. You can always go back later and try again.
- It helps to prepare before using these techniques. Think through your self-interview; perhaps even prepare some questions in advance. But don't try to anticipate where the session will go; that's injecting too much conscious thought into what should ideally be a spontaneous dialogue with your inner self or unconscious. You should know enough about yourself and your mind and body to have a sense of some possible causes for the problem and where the dialogue might go. Consider possible directions ahead of time.
- Stay flexible and spontaneous. Your session may end up going in a direction much different from the one you thought it would take. With the self-awareness exercise (3–A), go with the flow of your impressions. With the higher-level thinking exercise (3–B), keep asking gentle but probing questions after each answer until you get to the root cause. If you are unable to get any response at all, or the session simply goes nowhere, it's

likely eveidence of a deeply rooted negative emotion or limiting belief. Here are two suggestions if you get stuck:

1. Combine direct clearing techniques with pranic breathing (Chapter 4) and follow this with energy manipulation techniques, especially specific stress-reduction remedies that focus on cleaning out congestion from the solar plexus chakras (Chapters 9 and 13).
2. Try the mindfulness meditation (Chapter 11) for a while, and then go back and try these clearing techniques.

If neither of these solutions helps after a period of time, you may want to consider more traditional therapy with a professional who has experience in resolving emotionally based, physically manifesting health problems. You may want to consider one who specializes in hypnotism or bio-energetics.

Now, let's proceed with the exercises.

Trust Your Feelings and Impressions During These Techniques

"A few years ago I was working with a woman who had been referred to me for chronic bladder pain and urinary urgency and frequency. All traditional treatments had been ineffective. Using self-awareness, we had determined that she had been holding on to deep-seated anger, but we just couldn't identify the root cause, the precipitating incident in her past.

"After three sessions in which she insisted no insights had come to her during the awareness exercises, she decided to give up. 'Doc,' she said as she got up to leave, 'nothing's coming to me. I don't think it's working.' I asked her, 'Are you *sure* nothing at all came through? No visualizations or sensations that could account for your anger?' 'Nope, nothing,' she replied, 'except for this recurring image of my mother beating me and locking me in the closet. . . .'

"This was clearly the root cause we'd been looking for. But this woman didn't trust the image her unconscious had presented to her. She was unaware that her unconscious was communicating with her in this way, and she was uncomfortable acknowledging and feeling the truth of this admittedly very difficult memory.

"Listen to your body and accept the feelings, impressions, and images it presents to you."

—*Eric B. Robins, M.D.*

EXERCISE 3–A: *Clearing Negative Emotions and Limiting Beliefs with Self-Awareness*

This technique is most effective if you perform it when you can take time out of your schedule to be still and work quietly without interruption. A full routine is presented here. As you become more comfortable working with your inner self or unconscious, you can shorten parts of it—for instance, the relaxation part of the routine. Until you become familiar with it, however, take it step by step. You may wish to tape-record the directions so that you don't need to read the book at each step. This will give you a more complete relaxation.

1. Sit in a comfortable chair. You should be relaxed, and the room can be darkened. You don't want to be so relaxed or the room so dim that you fall asleep, however.
2. Close your eyes. Take eight deep breaths in order to relax further. Breathe slowly and deeply into your lungs.
3. It's easier to make contact with your unconscious mind if it is relaxed, and it's easier to relax your mind if your body is relaxed. So, begin by relaxing your body, one part at a time. You can work from the toes to the head, or from the head to the toes. Just be aware of each part for a few seconds, and say silently to yourself, "My (body part) is now completely relaxed." Breathe into the body part once, then breathe out, then let go. As you breathe, you can imagine inhaling relaxation into the area and exhaling tension from the area. Here is one physical relaxation sequence you might want to try:

1. Right foot and toes	12. Upper back
2. Right knee, leg below the knee	13. Right hand
3. Right thigh	14. Right wrist and forearm
4. Left foot and toes	15. Right elbow and upper arm
5. Left knee, leg below the knee	16. Left hand
6. Left thigh	17. Left wrist and forearm
7. Hips, pelvis, and buttocks	18. Left elbow and upper arm
8. Front abdomen	19. Neck and throat
9. Chest	20. Jaw
10. Lower back	21. Face
11. Spine	22. Head

Many find that this systematic relaxation exercise alone diminishes physical symptoms.

Self-Awareness Treatment for Functional Colitis

"A patient was referred to me with a nonurologic problem: intestinal spasms that his doctor had diagnosed as colitis, a functional disorder. Although he was taking Bentyl, an antispasmodic drug, to control his painful cramping, this man wanted to find the underlying cause of his problem. I had him close his eyes and led him through a progressive relaxation of his body. I then told him to trust whatever thoughts, sounds, images, or bodily feelings might arise as we conducted an internal scan of his body. As I had him focus on his colon, I asked him to remember the last time that he was having the spasms. When he could identify that, I asked him, 'What emotions were you experiencing at that time?' He instantly responded, 'Anger!' He had been having a dinner party at his house and felt that his wife was saying some inappropriate things that made him 'look bad' in front of their company. 'I felt a lot of anger toward her, and I felt upset at being stuck in a marriage with a person like her,' he continued. 'I've been having a lot of misgivings about my marriage, and a lot of anger, and I'm not sure what to do about it.'

"I asked him what he did when he felt these emotions of anger, and he said he did one of two things: either he suppressed the feelings since 'marriage is not supposed to be this way,' or he overate in order to mask his feelings. I told him that most people feel as if they only have two options to deal with anger: act out physically—yell at the person who is the presumed source of the anger, or attack them—or stuff the emotion deep in the body. I then explained that there was a third, more constructive option: to place objective awareness on the emotion and allow himself to feel the truth of what he was feeling. So we sat there, and he let himself feel angry at his wife for being 'stupid.' For the first time in his life, he acknowledged his anger and opened up to it. Not coincidentally, he also began to feel much more calm and peaceful. Shortly after this session, his colitis went away.

"He also learned to use self-awareness on his chronic lower back pain. Whenever he experienced a flareup of back pain, he would put himself in a relaxed state and place objective awareness on his back. As he sat still and aware, he would silently hold a thought, such as 'I wonder what I'm angry, fearful, or anxious about?' When the answer came to him, he opened up to it and allowed himself to feel those feelings. As he repeated this exercise, his back pain went away. It has been several years since he has had any recurrence of his back pain or colitis. Every time he feels an episode coming on, he does the awareness exercise, and gets in touch with what he is angry about, and lets himself feel his anger."

—*Eric B. Robins, M.D.*

4. In this quiet state, notice what you are feeling and where in your body you feel it. Breathe softly and quietly. Place your awareness on your entire body. Don't try to direct your awareness willfully to one part. If it is drawn to a particular area, fine. But don't begin with the thought that you want to be aware of your left foot or your head. Think of this as an internal scan of your entire body. Mentally note any sensations or impressions that arise as you become aware of your body. Spend about 5 minutes on this general scan.

5. Next, if you have a specific pain or ailment, put your awareness on the particular area or pain. If you have a headache, feel all the different feelings of having a headache. If you are experiencing abdominal discomfort, back discomfort, or even some emotional pain, put your awareness there. Gradually move your awareness deeper into the area or discomfort.

6. Be still, and notice what you are feeling. Stay relaxed, and be aware of any additional feelings or sensations that arise. Always trust the truth of what you are feeling or sensing. Be nonjudgmental. Don't make guesses or draw conclusions about why you are feeling or sensing certain things.

7. If you encounter resistance or feel an increase in the emotion or pain, or if you begin to feel heightened anxiety, this is your unconscious mind communicating with you. You are delving into an area that it has been protecting you from. Your unconscious has buried some negative emotion there. Keep your awareness there, if it's not too uncomfortable. Stay with the sensation; really be aware of it. Keep your breathing smooth and deep. (*Note:* If at any time the sensation or emotion becomes too intense or too uncomfortable, open your eyes and end the session. You can try again later.)

8. If you are focusing on a negative emotion or belief and you are able to stay with it, you should find it passing or diminishing in intensity within a short time. You should begin to feel some relief. It may be cleared away completely, or the relief may be only temporary. Perhaps it will return when you end the session. But when you go back in your next self-awareness session, you will have more knowledge. You work with the area again and emerge with a longer period of relief. And so on, until you are able to bleed away the negative emotion and clear it out of your energy body.

9. To end the session, thank your unconscious mind for its help, open your eyes, and slowly stretch before you get up and move around.

Higher-Level Thinking

The following story illustrates the principle of higher-level thinking. Two men were fishing on the side of a river one day. Suddenly, they heard some screams coming from the water.

They looked to the far side of the river bank and saw a woman struggling against the rapid current. One of the men jumped in to rescue her. The current was strong, and he was nearly pulled downstream himself. But with great effort, he managed to grab her and drag her to shore. She wasn't breathing, but they finally resuscitated her. By this time the other man had called 911 on his cell phone, and an ambulance had arrived, so they put the woman into the ambulance. Since they were now exhausted, the men decided to call it a day. As they were packing up their gear, they again heard screams from the water. They looked up to see two teenagers being swept along in the river, buffeted by the current and sharp rocks. The other man jumped into the river and again, after a heroic effort, pulled the two to safety. This time, the first man had called 911 and another ambulance had arrived. Almost immediately there were more screams coming from the water, and the fishermen saw two more people who seemed to be trapped in the torrent. The second man jumped in, saved the two and dragged them up onto shore, where they were put into a third ambulance. This pattern was repeated several more times: People struggled in the river, and the fishermen took turns pulling them out. What the men didn't see—nor did they think of looking for—was a crazed man a third of a mile up the river throwing people off a bridge.

Now, could these men have addressed the problem of drowning people in the river in another, more effective, way? They could have continued to rescue the people once they were already in the river, perhaps swimming faster and working more quickly. This would be working at the immediate level of the problem, which would be a time-consuming and ultimately unsuccessful approach. Or they could have strung a rope across the river to enable the people to catch on as they were swept downstream. This would be working with a little more creativity and at a little higher level. It would have enabled them to catch more people with greater efficiency and less effort, but doubtless, some people would still drown. Or, they could have worked at a much higher level, at its source, which would be preventing the crazed man on the bridge from throwing people over to begin with.

This story illustrates the basic premise of *higher-level thinking*: If you address a problem at a higher level—farther upstream, so to speak—you have quicker, more effective, and more lasting results.

Higher-level thinking is a more advanced form of self-awareness that helps you clear negative emotions, traumas, and limiting beliefs by engaging your unconscious mind in a dialogue, and then using nonjudgmental awareness to uncover the emotion, trauma, or belief that has been trapped in your body. There are seven steps in higher-level thinking:

1. Relax yourself physically and mentally.
2. Place nonjudgmental awareness on the problem.

3. Conduct a self-dialogue, using these four starter questions:

   "I wonder why (*this problem*) is occurring?"

   "What is (*this problem*) I'm having an example of?"

   "Why is this happening?" Or, put another way, "What is the higher purpose in my having (*this problem*)?"

   "What belief would I have to have in order to create (*this problem*)?"

4. Place light, nonjudgmental awareness on the affected area to see what negative emotions, traumatic memories, or limiting beliefs might be buried there that you have been trying not to feel.

5. Place nonjudgmental awareness on the uncovered emotion or trauma.

6. Feel the feeling, or the truth, of the emotion.

7. Let it go.

The centerpiece of this technique is the self-dialogue. Ideally, it should be a free-flowing give-and-take between your conscious and unconscious minds. As such, it is a conversation that is quite specific to each person and his or her problem(s), and thus, it's not possible to offer a standard "script" that every person can use. The four starter questions offered here, however, are the best that we've found to prompt that dialogue. The most effective approach is simply to practice the technique to become familiar with how to ask questions and how your unconscious mind responds (for example, an inner voice, a physical twinge, a sudden image). Begin the dialogue with one or more of the starter questions—or a question of your own that you derive from those questions—and go with the answers you get. Then pose follow-up questions that move you closer to the negative emotion, traumatic memory, or limiting belief that may be held in your body.

EXERCISE 3–B: *Clearing Negative Emotions and Limiting Beliefs with Higher-Level Thinking*

After you become more accustomed to working with your unconscious—understanding how it communicates with you in various ways—you can engage in higher-level thinking at any time: at work, at home, or while you're driving or waiting for an appointment. When you first begin to practice it, however, choose a time and place when you can be quiet and undisturbed, so that you can be fully relaxed. Take it step by step.

1. Begin with the same first three steps you used in Exercise 3–A: Sit comfortably in a chair, breathe deeply, and relax your body one part at a time.

2. As you are sitting relaxed and comfortable with your eyes closed, place your awareness on your health problem and the symptoms. (For this example, we'll use colitis.) Be lightly aware of the symptoms in the area of the body in which the problem occurs. Place your awareness on your stomach and abdomen. Maintain your objectivity. Try not to feel anxiety. Don't form any judgments. Don't blame yourself for having this problem, and don't become angry with yourself or conjure up the feeling that this is some type of fundamental weakness in your physical or emotional makeup. Simply become objectively aware of the symptoms or that part of the body. If you are experiencing cramping or bloating or any other symptom as you do this exercise, or if the symptoms start up as you do it, simply feel them, acknowledge them, and accept them, just as you did with self-awareness in Exercise 3–A. But don't dwell on any discomfort. Simply be with the discomfort; allow it to exist along with other feelings. Take your time doing this and continue to breathe deeply.

3. Now, silently form a question in your mind. Use one of the starter questions, or a question of your own derived from the starter questions. In the example we're using here, you could begin with, "I wonder why my intestines go into spasms. What might this problem be an example of?" Consciously hold the question for a few seconds, then relax, let it go, and return to your state of awareness and wait for an answer. Maintain a calm attitude of expectation as you wait; don't be too willful or demanding of your unconscious mind. Remember that the response can be verbal, visual, tactile, or symbolic. However the answers manifest, trust them.

4. The answer to one question leads to your asking another question and so on, until you get to the highest level of the cause for your problem. Let's assume you get this as your first response: "The smooth muscles in my intestines are clamping down." Thank your unconscious mind for the answer, then continue the dialogue. You might next ask, "Why would they be clamping down?" The answer might come back, "Maybe they're holding in an emotion or trauma that I have been unwilling or unable to face." As you hold nonjudgmental attention on the intestine, you might then wonder, "What specific emotions or trauma am I holding on to? Is it anger? Fear? Anger at what or whom? Fear of what or whom?" You might also want to check to see if you have any limiting beliefs attached to the problem, so you would ask at an appropriate point (and this *would* be an appropriate point), "What sort of limiting beliefs would I have to have in order to create this problem/these circumstances/block this healing energy?"

5. The answers from this point will move closer to the emotional root cause, so stay attentive and aware. You may get an answer quickly and surprisingly, or, you may need to probe deeper and ask additional questions. It is also possible that your unconscious mind

may get more protective and clamp down, so that no answer comes through at this time, or your physical symptoms worsen slightly. Aggravation of physical symptoms is almost always a sign that you are nearing an area from which your unconscious mind has been "protecting" you. If your mind suddenly goes blank, this is also usually a sign you are getting closer to the root cause.

6. If you get the answer, thank your unconscious mind and then place light, nonjudgmental awareness on the uncovered emotion, trauma, or memory for a while, as you learned to do in the self-awareness exercise. Be still, and notice what you are feeling. Stay relaxed and aware. Always trust the truth of what you are feeling or sensing. Feel the feeling, or truth, of that emotion, trauma, or memory, but don't be judgmental. Then let it go. You should find it passing or diminishing in intensity within a short time. As with self-awareness, perhaps the physical symptom or emotion will return later on, and you will need to do more sessions. With each session, though, you should feel the physical symptoms lessening and the emotional charge decreasing.

7. If you need to ask additional questions, keep probing until you get an answer or until you feel yourself tiring. If you feel like you're shutting down or getting tired before getting the answers you need or before 15 or 20 minutes are up, thank your unconscious mind for its help.

8. Open your eyes, and end the session. Slowly stretch before you get up and move around.

WESTERN MEDICINE IS NOT HIGHER-LEVEL THINKING

The story of the crazy man throwing people in the river also illustrates how standard medicine operates and why it often has difficulty addressing the ultimate cause of chronic, functional, or emotionally based ailments. *Standard allopathic medicine approaches health problems at the level at which they are occurring; it treats the symptoms.* Remember the traditional physician in the previous chapter who conducted a series of tests but found nothing wrong with his patient? He concluded there was little he could do aside from offering medications to alleviate the symptoms. His treatment plan is analogous to the fishermen pulling folks out of the river once they have already been thrown in. This physician was not looking upstream for the true higher-level cause. Nor are most physicians trained to look upstream for a higher-level emotional cause for ailments. Many health problems—and especially functional, recurring, or chronic health problems that have proven resistant to traditional medical interventions—can only be dealt with effectively by looking for the higher-level causes. That cause is ultimately energetic and, frequently, emotional.

Higher-Level Thinking for an "Inner Critic"

"I was working with a man who had a very tough 'inner critic,' a voice within that was constantly belittling him, saying things like, 'You're not good enough,' 'You'll never be a success,' and so on. During higher-level-thinking work, we asked a series of questions to get in touch with that critic to find out what its 'higher-level' intention was for him.

"After leading him through progressive relaxation and helping him place his objective, nonblaming awareness lightly on the voice, I had the man ask this critic what it was trying to do for him. The man suddenly experienced a tight sensation in his chest, then a flash of memory from childhood, from fifty years earlier, when he had been a brash, obnoxious, arrogant kid and quite unpopular because of his behavior. The man then had an abrupt insight: the 'purpose' of the voice was to keep him humble, so he wouldn't revert to his old ways. When we suggested to this 'critic' that perhaps it was time to be more loving and supportive because there was little danger of the man returning to those arrogant childhood ways, the man suddenly took a deep breath and felt the sensation in his chest disappear. At that moment, his inner critic left. It has not returned in nine years."

—*Eric B. Robins, M.D.*

CERTAIN CLEARING TECHNIQUES WILL WORK BETTER FOR YOU THAN OTHERS

After you have practiced the various clearing techniques, both direct and indirect, you likely will find that certain ones work better for you than others. Or you may find that one technique works well for a certain problem and another works better for another problem. For example, you may find, after you learn about pranic breathing in Chapter 4, that pranic breathing alone is very effective in clearing negative emotions and stress-related problems, but that higher-level thinking is more helpful in addressing deeper limiting beliefs or phobias. You'll read at the beginning of the next chapter the case of a woman who relieved anxiety caused by domestic problems simply through pranic breathing. However, a sixty-year-old woman plagued for years by headaches, nausea, agonizing bladder pain, and insomnia brought on by the limiting belief that she couldn't refuse to give money to irresponsible family members—despite her own meager income—needed to use self-awareness and higher-level thinking to get to the deeply seated root of her problem. (She had been beaten repeatedly as a child by her father for saying no, and thus, grew up believing she couldn't say no to anybody.)

You may also find that the energy manipulation techniques in Chapters 5 through 9 provide a quick, on-the-spot stress-reduction remedy, but that you need to supplement them with self-awareness to uncover the root cause of your stress reactions. Experiment a bit, then stick with what works for you. Don't try to master the entire range of techniques and apply all of them to all situations. Your goal is to have more energy and better health. You don't need to practice exercises that don't provide optimal results.

SIX STEPS DAILY PRACTICE ROUTINE

From this point forward, we will include at the end of each chapter a Six Steps Daily Practice Routine that includes suggestions for structuring your practice of the techniques. Each routine will incorporate your work up to that point and build on the routine from the previous chapters. In the beginning, when you're learning the fundamentals, try to practice for at least 15 to 20 minutes daily. As you progress and learn more techniques, your practice will become more individualized, depending on your needs, aptitude, and time available. You'll have many exercises from which to design your own program. Obviously, the more you practice, the faster you will develop, but don't feel you have to put in hours of training per day to get health and energetic benefits. Moderate, steady practice of about 30 minutes per day will produce excellent results.

Direct clearing techniques. Practice the direct clearing techniques—self-awareness and higher-level thinking, Exercises 3–A and 3–B—as needed, according to these guidelines:

- Either can be practiced daily, or even several times daily, until a problem is cleared and you no longer feel the negative emotion or limiting belief in your body.
- Each session should be 10 to 20 minutes long, depending on your ability to hold your attention and awareness productively and without strain.
- If you feel tired or uncomfortable before 20 minutes are up, simply end the session and try again later or the next day.

- Even if you have no issues that require work, it's valuable to practice direct clearing techniques to help you understand how your unconscious mind communicates with you.

In the next chapter, you'll learn the second of the six steps, *pranic breathing*. It's the simplest—yet perhaps the most powerful—of the techniques in this book.

CHAPTER 4
Take a Deep Breath— Pranic Breathing

"A few years ago I was going through some difficult times in my personal life. My body's reaction to this stress was my first anxiety attack, which left me completely out of control and feeling scared. The strange thing is that once my body reacted to stress with anxiety, it seemed to repeat that reaction every time I encountered stress. This reaction was so foreign to me that I immediately called my medical doctor, who referred me to a psychiatrist, who started me on Paxil and Ativan—a combination that was impossible for me to continue because I couldn't function at work or home. I also started seeing a therapist weekly, which helped but didn't stop these attacks. I knew Dr. Robins through work and confided in him how scared I was. He suggested I try a breathing technique called pranic breathing, which helped me instantly. I was so happy that the remedy was so simple and noninvasive. I could do these exercises at any time. I stopped taking the drugs, stopped paying my therapist a hundred and fifty dollars a week, and learned to breathe. It sounds so easy, and it is!"

—M.R., Los Angeles

Let's say your breathing is completely normal. You're inhaling and exhaling the average twelve or so breaths we draw into and push out of our 50 to 80 million alveoli (the tiny air sacs in our lungs that absorb the oxygen) each minute. Let's also assume that your breathing is unobstructed by problems such as allergies or asthma, and you don't smoke. In short, you're taking in all the oxygen you need to sustain life. You feel fine, and as far as you know, your breathing is fine. If someone asked you how your breathing was, you would likely tell them that it was normal. In fact, it would be normal.

But normal breathing is just "good enough" breathing. It's neither the best nor the healthiest way you can breathe.

While normal breathing is adequate for generating the baseline amount of energy needed to maintain daily life, it isn't sufficient to generate the quantity and quality of prana needed to make dramatic improvements in health. For that, you need to learn *pranic breathing,* the second of the six steps to self-healing. Pranic breathing can be learned in minutes. You can master it in days and feel its health benefits almost immediately.

THE TYPES OF BREATHING

Think of your lungs as divided roughly into thirds.

Clavicular breathing is breathing into the top third of the lungs and no deeper (Figure 4–1). Clavicular breathing is accomplished by raising the collarbone (clavicle) and shoulders during the inbreath and keeping the rest of the torso motionless. Clavicular breathing is the most shallow type of breathing. It brings oxygen into only the top third of your lungs.

Many women, particularly those who have had children, engage in clavicular breathing. Pregnancy makes it difficult for expectant mothers to breathe deeply, and the nine months of shallow breathing often ingrain the bad habit of breathing high and shallow even after childbirth. But many men are also clavicular breathers, particularly those who are overweight. Men with a "spare tire" have a slouching posture that inhibits deep breathing and they simply have never learned to draw breath any deeper into their lungs. In fact, many people take to smoking cigarettes partly because of the satisfying feeling that comes from pulling the oxygen—even more than the smoke—deeper into their lungs when they inhale. Pranic breathing can be an effective way to break the smoking habit.

Intercostal breathing is breathing into and filling the top third of the lungs, as in clavicular breathing, and then continuing to breathe into the middle part of the lungs (Figure 4–2).

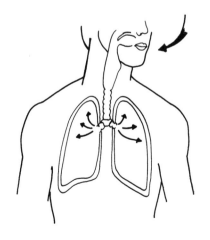

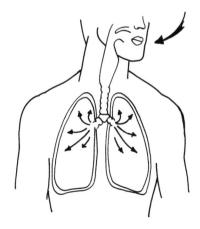

FIGURE 4–1   FIGURE 4–2

Intercostal ("between the ribs") breathing is accomplished by pulling up the clavicle, shoulders and torso, and then expanding the chest wall and ribs. Although many people breathe into their chests in this way, intercostal breathing is most common, and most easily seen, in athletes in the midst of competition. When you see a basketball or tennis player or anyone involved in an aerobic sport and their chest is heaving, that is an exaggerated form of intercostal breathing.

Diaphragmatic breathing is breathing into and filling the top two-thirds of the lungs and then breathing all the way down into the bottom third of the lungs (Figure 4–3). We also call this abdominal or pranic breathing. Abdominal breathing obviously does not mean that air enters the abdomen as you breathe, which is anatomically impossible. It simply means that as you breathe, you expand the abdominal muscles under the rib cage in the front and to the sides to permit the diaphragm to relax and move downward gently. Then, as the diaphragm lowers, you draw air deeper through the top two-thirds of the lungs and into the bottom third. Pranic breathing is a full, complete breath.

All living things have the inherent ability to assimilate prana during respiration. Even shallow breathing draws *some* air into all three portions of the lungs. A radiological test called a ventilation perfusion scan tracks the path of air as it is inhaled into the lungs and reveals that even people who are shallow breathers inhale a portion of air into the deeper part of the lungs. With pranic breathing, however, a greater proportion of inhaled air is drawn deep into the lungs, and a full, complete breath produces significantly more health and energetic benefits than shallow breathing.

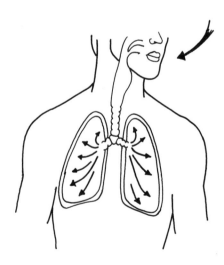

FIGURE 4–3

Why We Don't Breathe Properly

So, why don't we breathe properly? Why don't we automatically and unconsciously practice abdominal breathing without being trained to do it? Here are the main reasons:

- *Postural conditioning.* From an early age, we are taught to adopt a posture that is not conducive to abdominal breathing. In school, children are told to "stand up tall and straight." In the military, recruits are ordered, "Chest out, stomach in!" And modern paradigms of fitness and attractiveness emphasize an erect bearing, a flat stomach, and a curved-backward lower spine. All of these promote a posture that makes deep breathing difficult.
- *We hold negative emotions and tension in the muscles of the chest and abdomen.* Have you ever been so scared, angry, or stressed out that you felt like you couldn't breathe? As you read in Chapter 2, we frequently physicalize our stress and negative emotions; the unconscious mind traps them in the body. While this can happen in any part of our musculature, the chest and abdomen are prime sites for tightness, and the diaphragm muscle is particularly vulnerable. Tension held in the diaphragm manifests as a spasm or contraction, which makes it difficult to draw the diaphragm lower to take a deep breath.
- *Lack of awareness.* Many of us simply don't know we could breathe more deeply and more effectively and that deep breathing is healthier. We've been conditioned to breathe shallow and high, and we're unaware of how fully and powerfully we could breathe.

Abdominal breathing *is* normal breathing. If you doubt this, watch an infant asleep in a crib. As the child breathes, his abdomen moves in and out, slowly and rhythmically. You won't see the baby's chest, clavicle, or shoulders move as he breathes. It's not until we get older and more mature physically that social conditioning, stress, and tension inhibit our true normal breathing pattern.

Not only is abdominal or pranic breathing normal, in ancient esoteric spiritual traditions it has long been taught as the key to health and personal energy. Consider many traditional statues of the Buddha, which portray him with a soft, round, protruding belly. By contemporary standards of fitness and strength, which emphasize leanness and muscular definition, the Buddha is woefully unhealthy, but to energy and spiritual masters, the belly was a center of strength. A man with a belly such as the Buddha's could breathe deeply and powerfully and in so doing generate enormous energy to increase his personal health or spiritual enlightenment. These statues of the Buddha represent a person who knew how to breathe properly, a person with great energy and vitality.

THE BENEFITS OF PRANIC BREATHING

Pranic breathing delivers tremendous physiological and energetic benefits. The primary physiological benefits are:

- improved functioning of your waste-removal system;
- improved functioning of your cardiovascular system;
- a stronger, more supple diaphragm, which is good for your whole body and mind.

The primary energetic benefits include:

- an increased capacity for generating high-quality prana;
- indirect clearing of negative emotions, traumas, and limiting beliefs;
- an increase in the size of your spiritual cord. (Your spiritual cord is a thread that attaches your crown chakra to your higher self or soul. It is also the primary valve through which congested or dirty prana is expelled from the energy body and fresh prana is drawn into the energy body. Dirty prana, however, in addition to contaminating your overall energetic body, shrinks the diameter of your spiritual cord because it clogs this valve. Pranic breathing draws in a great amount of high-quality prana, which cleans out this valve and expands the size of your spiritual cord.)

To get a better understanding of how pranic breathing produces these benefits, let's first take a closer look at the internal geography of your torso, focusing on the diaphragm.

The diaphragm is a disk-shaped layer of muscle that bisects your chest cavity laterally (Figure 4–4). Attached to the bottom of the ribs and stretching backward and slightly downward to the lumbar vertebrae, it is quite flexible, but it is also one of the body's toughest and strongest muscles. The diaphragm acts as a divider between your cardiopulmonary system and your digestive system: it's the floor for your heart and lungs, and the roof for your stomach, intestines, spleen, liver, pancreas, and kidneys. As you can see from Figure 4–4, there's not a lot of room in your chest and abdomen; your organs are packed tightly. Thus when your diaphragm moves, it also moves your internal organs, giving them an internal massage. This is a good thing! Diaphragmatic movement stimulates the flow of blood and lymph into, through, and out of these organs in the chest and abdominal cavities.

A critical part of your immune system, lymph is a straw-colored fluid component of the blood that resembles plasma. It contains white cells but typically no red cells. As blood cir-

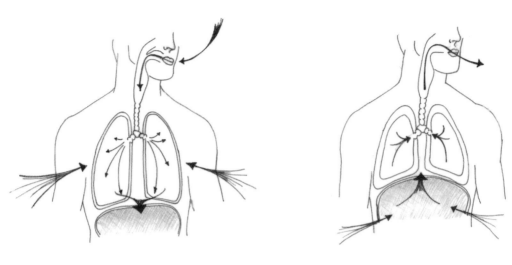

FIGURE 4–4

culates throughout the body, lymph separates from the blood, seeping out through blood vessels to bathe the body's tissues, where it picks up bacteria, waste products, toxins, and even random tumor cells. It then brings this cellular debris back to the lymph nodes, which are small round masses of lymphatic tissue located throughout the body. The lymph nodes break down this waste material and dispose of it. (The most commonly known lymph nodes are those in your neck along your jawline. If you have an upper respiratory infection, they may be inflamed, and the doctor may say you have "swollen glands.")

The lymph system, unlike the circulatory system, has no pump. Blood is forced through the body by the heart, but lymph must rely on muscular movement to facilitate its circulation. The arms and legs have many large muscles to move lymph. But throughout the chest, abdomen and pelvis, which contain numerous important lymph nodes in and around the organs, the only musculature available to help move the lymph fluid is the diaphragm. With this background, let's return to the benefits of pranic breathing.

Physiological Benefits of Pranic Breathing

1. *Improved functioning of your waste-removal system.* When you perform pranic breathing, your diaphragm relaxes and assumes a much greater range of motion than it does during shallower breathing. It moves farther downward into the abdomen on the inbreath and farther upward into the chest cavity on the outbreath. This down-and-up wave motion

of the diaphragm creates greater *negative intrathoracic pressure*, the suction effect that pulls lymph fluid up from the abdomen and pelvis into the chest, where it drains into the thoracic duct. From there it pours into one of the major veins running from the arm to the chest and then reenters the bloodstream, traveling to organs like the liver, spleen, and lungs to be cleansed. Pranic breathing helps move lymph through your organs and thus significantly improves your body's ability to detoxify itself.

2. *Improved functioning of your cardiovascular system.* Oxygenation is the process by which oxygen enters the lungs during inhalation and carbon dioxide leaves during exhalation. Pranic breathing increases oxygenation because it delivers more oxygen to the lower two-thirds of the lungs, which have a much richer flow of blood than does the upper third. The upper third of the lungs has a blood flow rate of one-tenth of a liter per minute, the middle third about two-thirds of a liter per minute, and the lower third about one to one-and-a-half liters per minute. The blood flow rate is the amount of blood moving through the lung tissue. Since the primary functions of the lungs are to get oxygen into the bloodstream and to carry away carbon dioxide from the bloodstream, it makes sense to get as much air as possible moving into and out of the parts of the lung where this is done most effectively. This is exactly what pranic breathing does. It helps your cardiovascular system function at peak capacity by increasing your intake of oxygen and reducing the strain on your heart.

3. *A stronger, more supple diaphragm.* As noted previously, we commonly hold tension, stress, and negative emotions in or near the diaphragm. A tight diaphragm can result in shallow breathing, an uncomfortably tight chest, and stomach spasms, which can interfere with digestion. Daily practice of pranic breathing and the torso-loosening exercises in this chapter help you stretch your diaphragm and release any tension you've accumulated there.

Energetic Benefits of Pranic Breathing

1. *An increased capacity for generating high-quality prana.* By combining pranic breathing with two techniques called *rhythm* and *retention* you significantly boost your energy-generation capability. Rhythm is breathing to a certain count, such as breathing in for an eight-count and out for a four-count, or using a five-count for both the inbreath and the outbreath. Different rhythms are used by different mind and body practices. Yoga, meditation, self-hypnosis, and martial arts all employ breathing rhythms, which help calm the body and clear the mind. A breathing rhythm shuts out external stimuli and con-

trols the chatter, self-talk, and random thoughts that run through your mind and prevent true relaxation. Thus, a breathing rhythm performs the same function as chanting or repetition of a mantra does during meditation: It focuses the attention. (A *mantra* is a word or sound repeated aloud or silently over and over while you meditate. The most well-known is the sound OM.)

Some breathing rhythms, however, do more than act as a focal point or pacing mechanism; they actually increase the amount of prana you draw in. When you combine the right rhythm with another powerful pranic breathing practice, retention, you can increase your energy-producing capacity tenfold or more with diligent practice.

Retention is purposefully holding your breath for a moment during the breathing cycle; it's the true secret to a massively energizing breath. Holding your breath after exhalation is empty retention and holding it after inhalation is full retention. Retention creates a pranic "bellows effect." Just as bellows are used to produce concentrated bursts of air to stoke a flame in a fireplace, rhythm and retention use a similar pumping effect to concentrate and magnify prana's natural cleansing and energizing effects within your body. Rhythm and retention also improve the distribution of prana, pushing it deeper and more forcefully throughout the body.

Here is how rhythm and retention work. During empty retention, when you compress the belly, deflate the lungs, and hold your breath for a moment, you create a physiological and energetic vacuum. It's comparable to pausing as you fully close a bellows before beginning to draw air in. When you begin your controlled inhale, as you draw oxygen into the lungs, you also pull tremendous amounts of prana into the pores and the chakras. You become highly energized.

During full retention, when your belly is completely expanded and you hold that full breath in your lungs, you're priming your energy pump. It's comparable to pausing just after you fully open a bellows before beginning to pump a blast of air into the fireplace. When you begin your controlled exhale, the energy is condensed and moves with greater force into the cells, organs, and chakras, where it is more fully and easily assimilated.

The right rhythm and retention are simple breathing adjustments, but they make a huge difference in the prana you are able to generate. In Pranic Healing classes, we do experiments to demonstrate the power of pranic breathing with rhythm and retention. We ask a person to stand in the front of the room and breathe normally, while a handful of students remain a few feet away on all sides and try to feel, or scan, the person's aura. Most people can feel it at about 6 inches all around the person's body. As the person begins pranic breathing, the students start feeling their hands being pushed back. If the person performs pranic breathing for as little as 3 minutes, it's not unusual for students to feel the aura expand to 20 feet or even more if the person is particularly strong. When we ask how the person who's breathing feels, invariably the reply is that he or she feels calm and powerful at the same time.

2. *Indirect clearing of negative emotions, traumas, and limiting beliefs.* As explained in Chapter 3, the mere act of breathing deeply from your abdomen may release tensions that you've been holding in your body, some of which you may not even be aware. This indirect clearing of negative emotions, traumas, and limiting beliefs can manifest in a number of ways: a wash of emotions that causes you to feel angry, sad, fearful, or anxious for no apparent reason; a sharp pain or spasm in some part of the body; or a trembling or shaking in some part of the body, to name just a few. These feelings can be unsettling, but they're normal. In fact, they are normal and good. They mean that you are releasing negative emotions and stresses that you've been holding onto. If you encounter these feelings, simply relax, and breathe through them as you learned in the self-awareness Exercise 3–A in Chapter 3. Be aware of the feeling without judgment or fear, then gently bring your awareness back to your breathing.

3. *An increase in the size of your spiritual cord.* You'll read more about your spiritual cord in the chapters on meditation and spiritual development, but the key to enlarging it is the retention step in pranic breathing, which cleans and expands the spiritual cord, thus permitting a larger supply of prana to enter the energy body more easily. Figure 4–5 shows a small, clogged spiritual cord and the dirty aura that results from it, while Figure 4–6 illustrates a clean, open spiritual cord and a pure, bright aura. When your spiritual cord opens up, you feel light and clean. Students who experience this opening report that it feels like a "huge waterfall of light" or a "warm feeling" pouring into their body.

PROGRESSIVE PRANIC BREATHING EXERCISES

You will learn pranic breathing in a three-stage progressive exercise routine:

1. Stretching and loosening your diaphragm
2. Pranic breathing
3. Rhythm and retention

As with all the progressive exercise routines, each level builds upon the previous one. The exercises are designed for you to follow in a specific order. You'll build a better energy

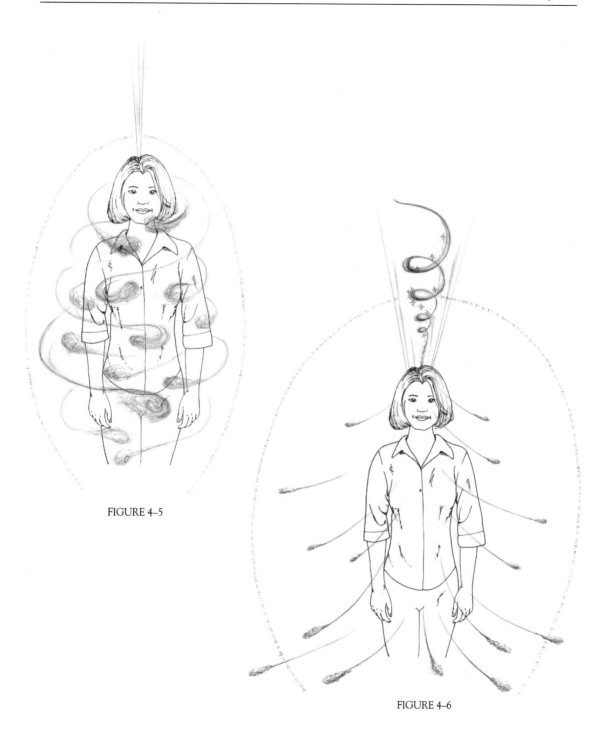

FIGURE 4–5

FIGURE 4–6

foundation if you perform them smoothly and properly at each level before moving on to the next level. But they are easy to perform, and you should move through the levels fairly quickly.

STRETCHING AND LOOSENING YOUR DIAPHRAGM

The following exercises stretch and loosen your diaphragm. They're from a set of *chi kung* exercises and will nicely supplement your pranic breathing practice. Even students with chronic tension in their torso or diaphragm report that they feel looser in less than two weeks of daily practice.

EXERCISE 4–A: *Stretching and Loosening the Diaphragm*

Pushing the Sky

1. Stand erect but relaxed with arms extended straight down in front of you. Your feet should be a shoulder-width apart.
2. Bend your wrists so that your palms face the floor. Then rotate your wrists inward 90 degrees so that the tips of your fingers are touching. Your elbows will also bow out slightly (Photo 4–a).
3. From this position, begin pranic breathing with a deep, slow inhale. As you inhale, swing your arms slowly upward in front of you in an arc. Keep your fingertips together and your elbows as straight as you can. Stop when your hands are directly above your head (Photo 4–b). You should still be holding your breath, and your palms should still be facing upward. At this point, push with your hands upward as if you are holding up the sky. You should feel light but real resistance. As you do this, you'll feel your entire rib cage and diaphragm pulled upward. Push for two to three seconds, relax, then exhale slowly as you let your hands separate and your arms float gently back to your sides (Photo 4–c). Time your exhalation so that it finishes as your hands arrive at your side.
4. Pause for one or two seconds, then bring the hands back to the starting position and begin again. As you do the exercise, try to begin to feel the energy inside you, especially when you are exhaling. With a little practice, you'll feel a cushion of energy under your hands as you lower them.

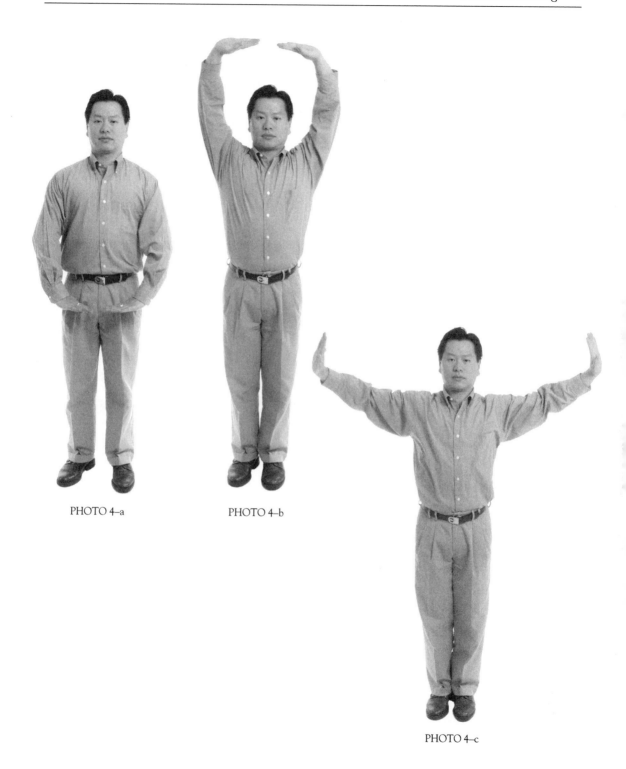

PHOTO 4–a

PHOTO 4–b

PHOTO 4–c

Looking at the Moon

1. Bend over at the waist, with arms and hands dangling loosely in front of you. Your knees can be straight, or if you have back problems, they can be bent slightly (Photo 4–d). From this posture, begin to straighten up and as you do so, begin your pranic breathing. As you inhale, lift and arc the arms straight up until they are directly over your head (Photo 4–e). Keep your arms and hands straight as you arc upward.

2. From this standing posture with your arms directly overhead, hold your breath, then arch backwards a few inches more. Curve your head and neck a bit more.

3. Form a triangle with your hands by touching your two thumbs and forefingers together. Then look through this triangle and imagine you are looking at the moon (Photo 4–f). After two or three seconds, straighten back up and exhale slowly while bringing your arms down to your sides. As with the first exercise, let them float down on the blanket or ball of energy. Really try to feel it.

Build up to eight repetitions of each exercise, and perform them before doing pranic breathing.

PRANIC BREATHING

Let's first feel the difference between clavicular or intercostal breathing and pranic breathing. You may perform this test standing or lying down, but if you're new to this breathing, it may be easier lying down because that posture will relax the diaphragm and abdominal wall more fully. Wear loose-fitting clothing, particularly around the waist. Lie on the floor, or on a mat or towel on the floor. Don't lie on a bed; a soft surface will cause your back to sag. Place one hand over your sternum or breastbone and the other below your navel, with your thumb directly on your navel. Now breathe as you normally do for about one minute. Most people will feel their chest, rather than their abdomen, move in and out. This is breathing high and shallow.

Now, in a seated position, let's learn to breathe from the abdomen.

EXERCISE 4–B: *Pranic Breathing*

(*Note:* Although all breathing and physical exercises in this book should be performed without strain, they do involve some effort. Check with your physician or medical adviser

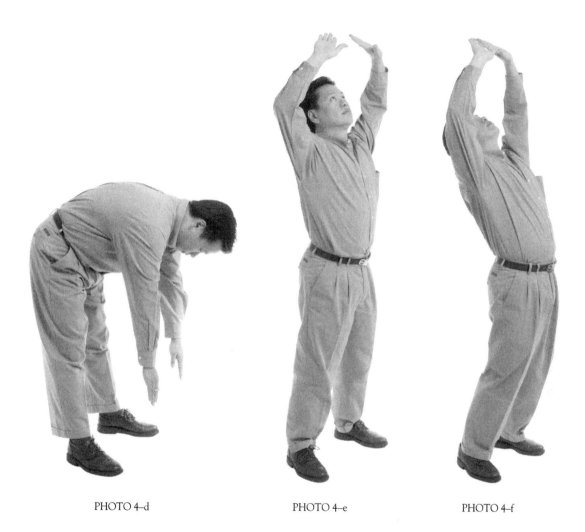

PHOTO 4–d   PHOTO 4–e   PHOTO 4–f

before starting this or any new exercise or breathing routine. If you have any preexisting health conditions, especially high blood pressure, migraines, or any type of heart or lung problems, get your physician's permission before beginning.)

1   Sit in a firm chair with your back straight. Move both hands to your belly, and rest your thumbs on your navel. You may find it helpful to close your eyes.

2.   Place your tongue on your palate and keep it there throughout the exercise

3.   Exhale through your mouth until your lungs are empty. Don't strain. Don't reach the end of your exhalation and then forcibly push out the air. Just exhale until your lungs are comfortably empty.

4.   With your mouth closed, breathe in slowly and silently through your nose. Feel the oxygen filling up first the top third of your lungs, then the second third and, finally, the bottom third. You should feel your abdomen push outward and downward. As your diaphragm flattens and the lungs open up, your hands should separate a bit, but your chest should not move. At the end of your breath, pause for a moment, then exhale. This is one cycle of pranic breathing. Don't worry for now about the count—that is, so many beats on the inbreath and so many on the outbreath. Repeat for up to ten times. Rest for a minute or two. Then try another set of ten breaths. See the Six Steps Daily Practice Routine at the end of this chapter for practice suggestions. (*Note:* Unless you are heavily congested or have chronic allergies, breathing through the nose is preferable to breathing through the mouth, for physiological rather than energetic reasons. The nose acts as a filter to keep small particles of dirt out of the lung and thus promotes cleaner breathing. Nasal breathing also warms up the air, which makes it easier to assimilate the prana.)

5.   There should be no strain. This isn't a competition to see how much air you can suck into your lungs. If you feel dizzy at all, stop and breathe normally for a few minutes.

Most people have the physical movement down within two weeks.

Help with Becoming Aware of Your Abdomen

If you have difficulty distinguishing between your belly and your chest moving during pranic breathing, the following exercise should help. It was developed by Gay Hendricks, Ph.D., and comes from his book, *Conscious Breathing: Breathwork for Health, Stress Release, and Personal Mastery.* Before you start, select a book that you can comfortably place on your stomach and still breathe easily. A hardcover book without the dust jacket is ideal; the rough binding helps keep the book from slipping off your stomach.

EXERCISE 4–C: *Keeping Your Focus on Your Abdomen Rather Than Your Chest During Pranic Breathing*

1. Lie down on your back on a firm surface.
2. Place a book on your belly over the navel area. The book should have enough weight that you can clearly feel it.
3. Place your tongue on your palate, and keep it there throughout the exercise.
4. Now, begin pranic breathing. Breathe slowly and deeply, making the book rise and fall on your abdomen with each breath. If you cannot make the book move, add more weight until you can clearly feel the area.
5. Be patient. When you begin to get breath into your abdomen, take away the book. If you lose the breath, put the book back.

Don't be put off by the simplicity of pranic breathing. While there are more dramatic techniques in this book, pranic breathing by itself has remarkable healing powers, as this story from Pranic Healing instructor Alejandro Armas demonstrates: "A friend was diagnosed with a blood disorder similar to lupus. I realized that her breathing was erratic, so I told her to start practicing pranic breathing every night. I also suggested that she imagine that she was inflating her belly as she was breathing in and that she was deflating it as she was breathing out. After several weeks of practicing pranic breathing, she noticed that she was not as tense, and she was sleeping much better. Then, when she went to her next check-up, the blood disorder was gone—much to her doctor's surprise. Since there was no medical cure for what she had and since the only thing she did differently was to practice pranic breathing regularly, we had to conclude that pranic breathing had relieved her of the disorder."

The "Master Breathing Technique"

"In one of my advanced study sessions with Grandmaster Choa, he told me that, in the ancient but little-known Jewish tradition of Kosher Yoga, the 7–1–7–1 method of breathing is known as the Master Breathing Technique. He then used this story to illustrate its power: Two men were walking down a quiet street when suddenly a mad dog rushed towards them. The first man became alarmed and yelled. The second man just calmly waved his hand in a brushing-aside gesture. The dog stopped in its tracks, turned around, and walked away. When the man who panicked asked what his companion did, the calm man said that he practiced the Master Breathing Technique, which allowed him to generate so much positive energy that he could deflect negative and violent energy."

—Master Stephen Co

RHYTHM AND RETENTION

After you have the physical movements of pranic breathing down, add these powerful rhythm and retention sequences. But one cautionary note before you begin: If you have high blood pressure, you should not hold your breath longer than one second. Although pranic breathing stimulates the navel, which is the body's primary storehouse of prana, it also stimulates the *meng mein* chakra, which is located opposite the navel on the back. As discussed in Chapter 1, the *meng mein* controls blood pressure. Thus, for people with hypertension, a longer breath retention could increase their blood pressure beyond their safety range.

EXERCISE 4–D: *Optimum Breathing Rhythm*

1. Place your tongue on your palate, and keep it there throughout the exercise.
2. Inhale for seven counts.
3. Hold for one count.
4. Exhale for seven counts.
5. Hold for one count.

This constitutes one cycle of pranic breathing with the 7–1–7–1 rhythm and retention sequence. Repeat steps one through five for each cycle. To begin your practice, perform three sets of 10 cycles, with a one-minute pause between sets. The entire practice should take you less than 10 minutes. (See also the Six Steps Daily Practice Routine at the end of this chapter.)

As you become more proficient at focusing on the breath, you internalize the rhythm, and won't need to be so aware of it or count it off in your mind. The length of the counts is not as important as maintaining the ratio and the steady pace. But a one-second-per-count rhythm is a good benchmark.

One of the best pacing techniques is to use a pulse count, timing your breathing and retention to your pulse. Using a pulse count also enables you to mark your progress, because as you become more experienced at pranic breathing and meditation, your pulse rate should slow down.

EXERCISE 4–E: *An Even More Powerful Retention Routine*

With this routine, the longer retention on both the inbreath and the outbreath stimulates the navel, *meng mein*, and basic chakras even more.

1. Place your tongue on your palate and keep it there throughout the exercise.
2. Inhale for *six* counts.
3. Hold for *three* counts.
4. Exhale for *six* counts.
5. Hold for *three* counts.

This constitutes one cycle of pranic breathing with the 6–3–6–3 rhythm and retention sequence. Repeat steps 1 through 5 for each cycle. As with the 7–1–7–1 sequence, perform three sets of 10 cycles, with a one-minute rest between sets. (See also the Six Steps Daily Practice Routine at the end of the chapter.)

In Pranic Healing classes, students scan each other while performing the two different breathing rhythm/retention sequences to feel the difference in energy-generation between them. "The energy definitely feels stronger for the 6–3–6–3," says Pranic Healing student Trish Sharpe. "It also feels more natural breathing in for the six-count and holding for three counts."

Continued pranic breathing compounds your ability to generate energy and helps you build a stronger energetic foundation, which enables you to generate a greater amount of prana with less effort in a shorter amount of time.

BREATH AS UNIVERSAL ENERGY NOT COMPLETELY ALIEN TO WESTERN CULTURE

Although the link between breathing and universal energy is more readily apparent in Oriental mind-body traditions, there is a Western esoteric breathing tradition, as well. It is even evident in our language. Consider the words *inspire* and *expire*, for instance. We use inspire today to refer to the act of motivating or encouraging ourselves or someone else to achieve an extraordinary goal, or to create something new and wonderful. But the word inspire comes from two Latin words: *in* (in) and *spirare* (to breathe). *Spirare*, in turn, is related to the Latin *spirit*. Thus, the word inspire was used in older times to indicate that someone was "breathing in spirit," or drawing in divine energy. Most frequently, it referred to an artist who was seeking guidance on the creative process, or a holy man seeking energy for prayer or healing.

The primary definition of *expire* today denotes the end of a period of time—for instance, the completion of a politician's time in office (term expired), or the date beyond which a food product is no longer safe to eat (expiration date). But we also use the word to connote the end of life: A person who has expired has breathed out his last breath. As the breath leaves, so does the life force.

A Few Notes on Pranic Breathing

- There's an old Chinese martial arts saying that's translated roughly as "smooth is fast." This maxim is drilled into beginners who attempt to build up speed and power in their fighting techniques by using too much effort and trying too hard. The true way to attain proficiency—in any new endeavor or skill—is to focus on being smooth and controlled rather than exerting a "110-percent effort." The same principle applies to your pranic breathing practice. Like most aspects of the energetic routines in this book, pranic breathing isn't a conscious or willful process. In fact, concentrating in a lips-pursed, fists-clenched way is counterproductive to relaxed, smooth pranic breathing. When you're learning a new skill, however, it's normal to focus on the mechanics until they become second nature. Thus, you may find yourself consciously repeating the count: "Inhale 1, 2, 3, 4, 5, 6, 7, hold 1, exhale 1, 2, 3, . . . " along with other instructions. In the beginning, feel free to focus on performing the technique correctly, making sure you have the right count, keeping your chest still, and so on. But check yourself after a week or two to make sure that your pranic breathing is becoming smooth. If it takes a little longer than two weeks, that's fine, but practice until pranic breathing happens with the right rhythm and retention without your thinking about it.
- Effective pranic breathing is deep, purposeful—and slow. If you need help slowing down your breathing, the number one tip is, don't *consciously* try to slow down. Avoid making pranic breathing a willful effort. Don't tell yourself, "slow down, slow down, slow down." If you must think about something in the early stages of your training, think about the mechanics of pranic breathing, such as making sure you are moving your diaphragm fully down and up and that your belly is moving and your chest isn't. As you progress, gradually allow yourself to let go and be drawn into your pranic breathing practice. It will eventually become second nature to you.

PRANIC BREATHING CHECKLIST

1. Wear loose-fitting clothing, particularly around the waist.
2. Close your eyes and relax your body.

3. Become aware that you will be taking a full, complete breath. You are going to fill up your entire lungs.

4. Place your tongue on your palate, and keep it there throughout the exercise.

5. Begin by breathing out through your mouth gently until your lungs are comfortably empty.

6. With your mouth closed, breathe in slowly and silently through your nose.

7. Feel the top third of your lungs fill up, then the middle third, and finally the bottom third. Your chest should not move as you inhale. Your abdomen should push out in the front and a little on the sides as you breathe in. Place your hands on your belly and your thumbs on your navel as needed for reinforcement.

8. Pause for a moment (full retention).

9. Slowly begin your controlled exhale. Feel the air vacate your lungs, first the lower third, then the middle third, and finally the upper third.

10. Pause for a moment (empty retention), then begin another inhalation.

SIX STEPS DAILY PRACTICE ROUTINE—UPDATE

1. *Direct clearing.* Practice the direct clearing techniques (Exercises 3–A and 3–B, self-awareness and higher-level thinking) as needed, according to the checklist at the end of Chapter 3.

2. *Stretching, loosening the diaphragm.* Build up to eight repetitions of each part of Exercise 4–A. Use them prior to pranic breathing, or until you feel your torso and diaphragm loosen up.

3. *Pranic breathing.* Do three sets of ten pranic breaths (Exercise 4–B). If necessary, begin with your hands on your belly with your thumbs on your navel to feel the abdomen move in and out. Progress to the 7–1–7–1 and then 6–3–6–3 rhythm and retention sequences.

In the next five chapters, you'll learn the third of the six steps to self-healing, the *energy manipulation techniques* of scanning, sweeping, and energizing. It begins in Chapter 5 with scanning.

Hands Up! Scanning— Hand Sensitivity and General Scanning

"A relatively new Pranic Healing student came to class complaining of edginess, irritability, anxiety, and exhaustion. He said he had no medical problems but was under a lot of pressure at work and at home. I performed general scanning of his aura from all sides and found several areas of congestion and depletion, the most significant of which was a seriously congested and overactivated meng mein chakra. Its energy protruded several feet from his body. The meng mein controls, among other things, the body's overall vitality, the adrenal glands, and blood pressure. Three of the most common physical symptoms of stress are fatigue, overstimulation of the nervous system due to excessive adrenaline in the body, and elevated blood pressure."

—DANIEL O'HARA, MISSION VIEJO, CALIFORNIA

How can you sense the shape of your energetic anatomy and the size of your chakras? How can you know when there is an energetic disturbance in the aura? How can you detect when pranic breathing with rhythm and retention has doubled the size of your aura or increased your ability to generate prana tenfold? One way would be to be born with a heightened awareness of energy, which would enable you to sense or see the aura and the energetic changes in it. There are people who have this ability naturally. Another would be to take special training to help you cultivate heightened visual acuity to this subtle energy. Grandmaster Choa utilized people with a sensitivity to energy—some of whom were born with the skill, others who developed it through training—in his original experiments to develop the Pranic Healing system. But a third, easier, and quicker way to detect changes in the aura is to learn *scanning*, which is the ability to feel the contours and strength of energy aura. Scanning is a heightened sense of touch and requires only that you sensitize the palm chakras in the center of your hands.

Scanning is the first of three *energy manipulation* techniques that will enable you to perform healing work directly on your aura. *Energy manipulation* is the third of the six steps to self-healing. You will use scanning in three ways:

1. to feel your energetic anatomy for any disturbances that may indicate a health problem;
2. to measure your progress in generating prana by feeling the increase in your own energy as you perform the exercises;
3. to get tactile energetic feedback to reinforce your practice.

PROGRESSIVE SCANNING EXERCISES

Scanning may sound mysterious, but it's actually easy to learn. Chapters 5 and 6 contain seven levels of progressive exercises to help you acquire this skill:

Chapter 5

1. Developing hand sensitivity
2. General self-scanning
3. Scanning other life forms: plants and animals
4. Scanning another person

Chapter 6

5. Specific self-scanning
6. Scanning using visualization
7. Interpreting your results

These exercises follow a logical sequence, with each level building upon the previous one. The first four levels, presented in this chapter, include drills to help you develop the hand sensitivity you need to perform *general self-scanning*, which is feeling the overall strength of your aura. The final three levels, presented in Chapter 6, include exercises for *specific self-scanning*, which is a more targeted scanning of chakras and specific areas in your aura. Chapter 6 also teaches you how to interpret your scanning results.

It usually takes no more than two weeks of daily practice, about 15 minutes a day, to learn to scan. It may take a little longer, but once you get the feeling of the energy, your hands are more or less permanently sensitized. Even if you can't perform the exercises at one or more of the levels—for instance, if you don't have appropriate plants or animals on which to practice, or a partner with whom you can work—you can still learn to scan. Just spend more time on the levels you *can* do by yourself, such as hand sensitivity and self-scanning.

As in the progressive pranic breathing exercise sequence in Chapter 4, try to spend sufficient time on each level before moving on to the next, so that you build a good foundation for your energy sensitivity. It's better for your development if you're sure that you can really feel the energy in the hand sensitivity exercises before you move on to general scanning of your body and the other scanning techniques. As we pointed out in Chapter 1, though, even if you can't feel the energy, simply continue with your practice. If you feel you're stuck at one level and can't feel the energy, just move on to the next exercise. Even if you're not sure you're feeling prana by the time you get to the healing routines in Chapter 13, you can still perform them and make them work for you.

DEVELOPING HAND SENSITIVITY

Hand sensitivity exercises open the hand chakras and enable you to feel your prana. You're already familiar with the hand chakras because the first exercise you did in Chapter 1, Detecting Your Energetic Anatomy (Exercise 1–A), is really Hand Sensitivity Exercise 1. You will use that exercise or Exercise 5–A or both as part of your regular practice.

EXERCISE 5–A: *Hand Sensitivity Exercise 2*

Stand comfortably while performing this exercise.

1. Put your tongue on your palate.
2. Perform a few cycles of pranic breathing to clear and calm your mind and relax your body.
3. Tap your heart chakra several times with any two fingers of your scanning hand. For most people, the scanning hand is the dominant hand. The heart chakra is located in the center of the chest, directly between the nipples. Since the heart is the seat of sensitivity, tapping your heart chakra heightens your ability to sense and feel subtle energy.
4. Wrist rolls: Extend your arms straight out in front of you at shoulder height. With your hands open and your fingers relaxed, roll your hands at the wrists 10 times in both directions; make small circles with your hands pivoting at the wrist, stirring 10 times clockwise and 10 times counterclockwise.
5. Hand openers: Open and close your hands vigorously 10 times.
6. Elbow, finger shake: Begin with your arms at your sides. Bring your fists up near your

shoulders as if you were curling up a dumbbell in your hands. The back of your hands should be facing away from you. From this position snap your arms down.

7. Without jarring your elbows, flick your fingers open as you reach the bottom as if you were dropping the imaginary dumbbells, and then back up 10 times quickly.

8. With the thumb of your right hand, press down lightly into the center of your left palm for a few seconds. Then repeat the movement with your other hand, using your left thumb to press down into your right palm.

9. Raise your right hand above your head and push up with your palm, while at the same time moving your left hand down and pushing down with that palm (Photo 5–a). Exert light pressure upward and downward for a few seconds, but don't tense your muscles.

10. Reverse the hand position, pushing up with your left palm and down with your right (Photo 5–b).

11. Repeat these hand pushing movements two more times.

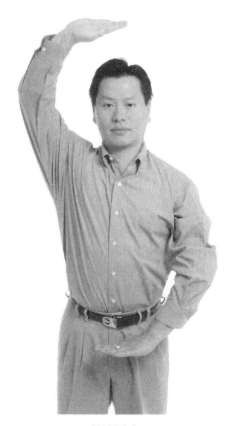

PHOTO 5–a

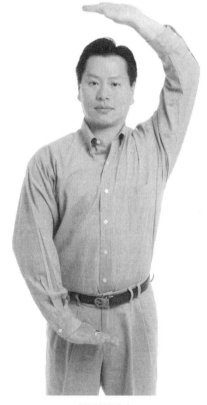

PHOTO 5–b

12. Stretch your hands in front of you, with your palms about 3 inches apart and facing each other as if you were about to clap your hands. Keep your forearms extended in front of you and parallel to the ground. Keep your hands relaxed and your armpits open. It's the same posture you used in Exercise 1–A (Figure 1–4). Close your eyes. Keeping your hands a few inches apart, just breathe slowly and focus lightly on the centers of your palms. Do this for about 10 seconds.

13. Then, keeping your hands, wrists, and elbows steady, begin to move your arms in and out a few inches from each other, moving your hands closer together and then farther apart. Pretend you are clapping your hands in very slow motion, but don't let your hands meet. Bring your palms to within an inch or two of each other and then, slowly, move them out about a foot. Then, bring them close together again. Repeat this action until you feel the prana between your hands.

Don't worry if you don't feel anything. If you don't sense a warm, itchy, or tingling sensation in your palms after completing this exercise once, stop for a few moments, perform a few cycles of pranic breathing, focus on your palms again, and do the exercise again. If you lose contact or sensitivity, take a break and perform more pranic breathing exercises or try Hand Sensitivity Exercise 1. You'll feel the energy before too long.

What If You Still Can't Feel the Energy?

If you still can't feel the energy as you do the Hand Sensitivity Exercises, relax. Stick with your practice; you'll feel it. Keep a positive attitude and an open mind. Doubts, fears, and apprehensions inhibit your ability to sense and manipulate subtle energy. If you attempt to sensitize your hands while thinking, "this isn't working," or "this is weird," you will have a more difficult time. Control your thoughts, but don't try to fool yourself into feeling something that isn't there. The energy is not imaginary; it's real, and you *can* feel it using these exercises. So don't imagine or anticipate that you're feeling energy if you're not. With steady, regular practice, anyone can develop the ability to feel the energy, as Pranic Healing student Arnon Davidovici found out. "For about six months after taking Pranic Healing, I would always rationalize away or second guess anything I felt during scanning," he reports. "The day I really started to feel prana was the day that I decided to accept the first thing I felt. I was not always 100 percent accurate, but I decided that that was okay because I was still learning. Over time, my accuracy has improved. I now feel pressure or a flow of energy when scanning. If the energy is dirty, it usually feels itchy, tingly, and sometimes sticky or heavy. If the energy is particularly high vibration it can feel tingly (but not itchy), or it can have a smoothness to it like light, soft cream."

Here's a tip from our classes: People who pick up scanning very quickly in class use positive reinforcement to accelerate their development. As soon as they feel any sensation at all, they tell themselves that what they are feeling is prana and that they are doing well. They put the critical part of their mind aside and use positive self-talk to reinforce that they are feeling the energy. Whenever they detect a feeling, they use positive self-reinforcement to help them learn scanning more quickly.

GENERAL SELF-SCANNING

General self-scanning is feeling your aura at various points to get a sense of its overall strength and cleanliness. In this first exercise, you will scan your arm, just because it's an easy target for beginners.

EXERCISE 5–B: *General Self-Scanning of Your Arm*

You may sit or stand as you do this exercise. *Note*: As you progress, we will shorten the description of the warm-up steps. Also, we presume you scan with your right hand and that your left forearm is the scanning target. But reverse the directions if you're scanning your right forearm with your left hand.

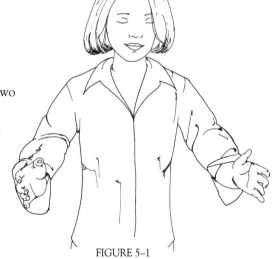

1. Place your tongue on the roof of your mouth.
2. Perform a few cycles of pranic breathing.
3. Tap your heart chakra several times with any two fingers of your scanning hand.
4. Perform Hand Sensitivity Exercise 1 or 2 until you can clearly feel the energy between your hands.
5. With your elbows bent at a 90-degree angle and your forearms in front of you roughly parallel to the ground, extend both hands in front of you, waist high, as if you were holding a large beach

FIGURE 5–1

ball in front of you. Your palms face each other. Your arms, hands, and fingers should be relaxed. Your fingers should be slightly separated, your hands and wrists loose, and your armpits open; your arms should not be pinned to your sides. Your arms should be about 3 feet apart (Figure 5–1).

6. When you scan, you need to tune in to your target, to establish your *intent* to scan. You do this by looking briefly at your scanning target for a few seconds and then declaring your intent silently to yourself. Example: "I now intend to scan (whatever it is that you intend to scan)." Since your scanning target for this exercise is your left forearm, look at a spot on the inside of your left forearm for a few seconds, and then say to yourself, "I now intend to scan my left forearm."

7. Once you've established your intent, turn your awareness to the palm chakra of your scanning hand, and keep your awareness there as you scan. Remember the concept of awareness from Chapter 2. Awareness is not concentration, nor is it intense staring or even watching; it's not a visual sense. Rather awareness is a quiet, soft, still but active sensing. It's a feeling of heightened sensitivity. In scanning, you are *feeling* the energy rather than seeing it. Keeping your awareness focused on your scanning hand heightens the sensitivity of your hands to this subtle energy.

8. Your concentration level when you scan should be about the same used in reading a book. Don't tense up and try to force yourself to scan. The type of awareness used in scanning is best achieved with a light focus but not a high degree of will. Trying to impose your will in scanning inhibits sensitivity.

9. Breathe slowly and deeply, using pranic breathing.

10. Keep your eyes open or closed. (As you become more proficient, you can scan with your eyes open, but in the beginning, in order to not be distracted, you may find it helpful to scan with your eyes closed.)

11. Keep a positive, open-minded attitude.

12. From the holding-a-beach-ball position, begin scanning by moving your right hand slowly toward your left forearm. Scan horizontally directly across the front of your body (Figure 5–2). Do not move

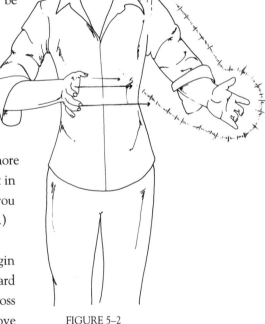

FIGURE 5–2

your left arm. Keep the fingers of your right hand in a natural, relaxed position— slightly curved and open. Slow down more as your right hand gets about a foot away from your left forearm. Now move your right hand forward and back within a range of 4 to 12 inches from your left forearm, as if you were lightly feeling it from afar, which is exactly what you are doing. You are feeling for your body's energy field, like very lightly feeling the surface of a perfectly calm pool of water. Keep breathing slowly and deeply. Your right hand should neither touch nor move more than a foot away from your left forearm. Keep your awareness on the center of the palm of your scanning hand. Keep the joints of your shoulder, elbow, wrist, and hand loose and supple as you move your scanning hand forward and back.

13. Stop your hand when you get a feeling of pressure, tingling, itchiness, or heat in your palm. You should feel this sensation as you get within 4 to 10 inches or so of your left forearm. This is the inner aura, the area where you will do most of your healing work.

14. If you don't feel the energy right away, don't be discouraged. Simply relax, breathe deeply, and move your right hand back from your left forearm and then in again until you feel it. If after 10 to 12 movements you still have difficulty feeling the energy, repeat Hand Sensitivity Exercise 1 or 2, or tap your heart chakra again.

15. If you continue having difficulty feeling the energy, try scanning in from another angle. Begin with the holding-a-beach-ball position, then raise your right hand to about shoulder level. Scan downward at a 45-degree angle, or lower your right arm to a point below your waist and scan upward. The angle you take in scanning is unimportant. Whichever angle you take, though, make sure you begin scanning about 3 feet away from your target.

16. When you feel pressure, tingling, or warmth in your scanning hand, notice how far away your scanning hand is from your forearm. Is it 6 inches away? Two inches? Eight inches? This is the *depth* of your aura, how far your energy aura extends out from your physical body. Most adults in a state of general well-being have an aura that radiates out from the body about 5 inches. If you find that your aura is deeper or more shallow than 5 inches, don't worry. For now, simply take note of the depth of your aura. For very specific reasons, we hold off discussion of what these scanning measurements mean until we get to Chapter 6. You may want to jot down your results so that you can refer to them later.

17. Try to sense the strength of the aura as you continue to move your hand forward and backward. Do you feel a strong sense of pressure or tingling? Does it feel like your hand is being repelled forcefully? Or do you feel only slight pressure?

18. Conclude the exercise by walking around for a few minutes and shaking your arms and legs. Relax and take a few deep breaths.

After you've finished, you may want to jot down your scanning impressions so that you can refer to them later.

Using this same sequence, now scan a few other parts of your body: another point on your arm, various points on your legs, and so on. As you do, try to sense the depth and strength of your aura at different points. You may wish to jot down these scanning impressions, too.

What If You Still Can't Feel the Energy?

If you don't feel your energy during this exercise, even after trying all the alternatives, you may wonder if you have a relatively weak aura. This is possible, but it's more likely that, at this stage of your scanning development, you haven't developed sufficient sensitivity. If you have difficulty feeling your aura in this exercise, don't worry. You will develop the ability with practice. See the Six Steps Daily Practice Routine and the Scanning Checklist at the end of this chapter.

SCANNING OTHER LIFE FORMS: PLANTS AND ANIMALS

Exercises for scanning plants and animals are included in a self-healing routine simply because they provide good practice. Their energetic anatomy is different from a human's, but they can help you build the skill of feeling life force.

EXERCISE 5–C: *Scanning a Plant*

Choose a good, healthy plant so that you are working with a vibrant energy aura. Any thriving tree, flower, or plant will do, but some are particularly good: small pines, most citrus trees, Hawaiian *ti* plants (also known as "good luck plants"), ficus, and spider plants, to name a few. Avoid desert plants such as succulents and cacti. Their energy aura is irregular, prickly, or sharp due to their shape, and may be difficult for beginners to detect.

Stand for this exercise. You should be familiar with the four-step warm-up: Place your tongue on the roof of your mouth. Perform a few cycles of pranic breathing. Tap your heart chakra several times with any two fingers of your scanning hand. Perform Hand Sensitivity Exercise 1 and/or 2 until you can clearly feel the energy between your hands.

1. Stand about 3 feet away from the plant with your scanning arm, hand, and fingers relaxed.

2. Look at a portion of the plant to tune in to your target. Pick a specific limb, leaf, or flower and form your intent to scan the aura at that spot.

3. Remember: Breathe slowly and deeply, using pranic breathing. Keep your awareness on the palm chakra of your scanning hand. Once you have looked at the plant to establish your intent, keep your awareness on your scanning hand throughout the rest of the scanning exercise. Keep a positive, open-minded attitude.

4. Begin scanning by moving your hand in slowly toward the plant or tree from about 3 feet away (Figure 5–3). The angle of approach that your scanning hand takes is unimportant. You can scan in from the side, from above the plant downward, or from below the plant upward.

5. Breathe slowly and deeply. Move your scanning hand in carefully, in that steady forward-and-back motion. Take your time.

6. Stop when you get that feeling of pressure, heat, tingling, or resistance. Depending on the type and health of the plant you are scanning, you should feel the aura at 4 to 10 inches from the plant. Move your hand backward and forward a few times. Note how far out the aura extends. Once you definitely feel the energy, get a sense of its relative strength.

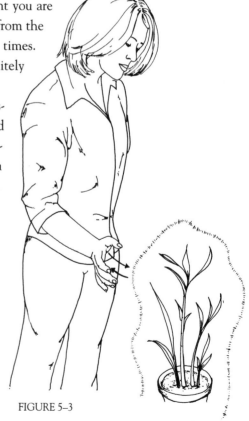

7. If you don't feel the energy right away, don't be discouraged. Relax, breathe deeply, and move your hand back and then in again until you feel it. If after 5 minutes you still have difficulty feeling the energy, take a few minutes and repeat Hand Sensitivity Exercise 1 or 2, or tap your heart chakra again.

8. Now scan the plant from different angles, from above and below your initial scanning point and from another side. See if you can detect the overall shape and strength of the plant's energy aura. Is it uniform on all sides? Does the aura feel 5 inches deep all the way around, or does one side or area feel more shallow than the other? Does it feel relatively strong or weak?

9. Conclude the exercise by walking around for a few minutes and shaking your arms and legs. Relax and take a few deep breaths.

FIGURE 5–3

After you've finished, you may want to jot down your scanning impressions so that you can refer to them later.

You may find it helpful to practice scanning different plants, flowers, and trees to see which have the strongest auras. Jot down these scanning impressions for comparison with your first effort.

EXERCISE 5–D: *Scanning an Animal*

As with the plant exercise, it's best to practice on an animal that you know is in good health. A strong aura is easier for beginners to detect. Dogs and cats are good subjects because they are the most common animals available to us and because they sleep frequently, which gives you a chance to practice on a willing subject.

Perform the four-step warm-up, then proceed.

1. Sit, stand, or even kneel, if your animal is sleeping on the floor, a few feet away from the subject with your scanning arm, hand, and fingers relaxed.

2. Look at the animal to tune in to your target. Pick a spot—say, the shoulder, hip, head, or belly—and form your intent to scan the aura there.

3. Breathe slowly and deeply, using pranic breathing. Keep your awareness on the palm chakra of your scanning hand. Once you have looked at the animal to establish your intent, keep your awareness on your scanning hand throughout the rest of the scanning exercise. Keep a positive, open attitude.

4. Beginning with your scanning hand about 3 feet away from the animal, move your hand in slowly from whichever angle you prefer. Scan toward your targeted spot (Figure 5–4).

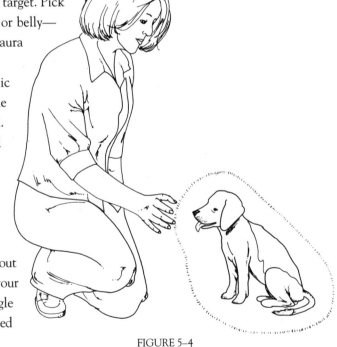

FIGURE 5–4

5. Breathe slowly and deeply. Move your scanning hand in carefully, in that steady forward-and-back motion.

6. Stop when you get that feeling of pressure, heat, tingling, or resistance. Depending on the type and health of the animal you scan, you should feel the aura somewhere in the range of 4 to 10 inches from the animal. Move your hand backward and forward a few times. Note how far out the aura extends. Once you definitely feel the energy, get a sense for its relative strength.

7. If you don't feel the energy right away, don't be discouraged. Relax, breathe deeply, and move your hand back and then in again until you feel it. If, after 5 minutes, you still have difficulty feeling the energy, take a few minutes and repeat Hand Sensitivity Exercise 1 or 2, or tap your heart chakra.

8. Then, as with the plant, scan a few different locations on the animal's body and from different angles. See if you can detect the overall shape and strength of the animal's energy aura. Is it uniform on all sides? Does the aura feel 4 inches deep all the way around, or does one side or area feel more shallow than the other? Does it feel relatively strong or weak?

9. Conclude the exercise by walking around for a few minutes and shaking your arms and legs. Relax and take a few deep breaths.

After you've finished, you may want to jot down your scanning impressions so that you can refer to them later.

Again, as with plants, if you have access to different animals, you may want to scan them to see which have the strongest auras. Jot down these scanning impressions for comparison with your other scanning efforts.

Pranic Healing student and energy healer Tiffany Cano, who has both people and pets as clients, notes that the auras of animals tend to be about the same depth as those of humans, depending on the animal's level of vitality. She also reports that animals' chakras are located in the same general area as humans', but they tend to be proportional to the animal's size and thus smaller than human chakras.

SCANNING ANOTHER PERSON

The mechanics used in general scanning of another person are no different from those used in general scanning of a plant or animal. Your goal is the same: to get a sense of the overall strength of the aura. The only difference is that this subject can provide verbal feedback on any specific problems that you may sense during your scan. But ask him or her not to respond until after you've finished your scan, even if you comment on where you think you feel energetic disturbances in the aura.

EXERCISE 5–E: *Scanning Another Person*

For this exercise, it is better if you stand. Your subject can sit or stand. He should just relax and breathe naturally. He can keep his eyes closed if he wishes. He should keep his tongue on the roof of his mouth to increase sensitivity. Perform the four-step warm-up, then proceed.

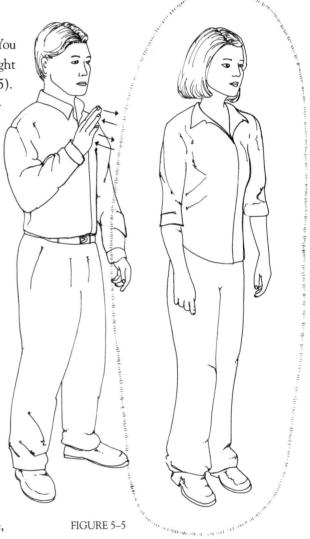

1. Stand 2 to 3 feet away from your subject. You should be off to the side rather than straight in front of or in back of him (Figure 5–5). You will scan the upper arm area (anywhere between the shoulder and the elbow). The arm, hand, and fingers of your scanning hand should be relaxed.

2. Look at your target to tune in and form your intent to scan.

3. Breathe slowly and deeply, using pranic breathing. Keep your awareness on the palm chakra of your scanning hand. Once you have looked at your target to establish your intent, keep your awareness on your scanning hand throughout the rest of the scanning exercise. Keep a positive, open-minded attitude.

4. Beginning with your scanning hand about 3 feet away from your subject's body, move your hand in slowly from whichever angle you choose toward your target spot. Breathe slowly and deeply. Move your scanning hand in carefully.

5. Stop when you get that feeling of pressure,

FIGURE 5–5

heat, tingling, or resistance. You should feel it as you get within 4 to 10 inches of the person. Remember, the average healthy adult has an inner aura that's about 5 inches deep. Move your hand backward and forward a few times. Note how far out the aura extends. Really feel it. Once you definitely feel the energy, get a sense of its relative strength.

6. If you don't feel the energy right away, don't be discouraged. Relax, breathe deeply, and move your hand back and then in again until you feel it. If after 5 minutes you still have difficulty feeling the energy, take a few minutes and repeat Hand Sensitivity Exercise 1 or 2, or tap your heart chakra.

7. Scan a few different locations and from different angles. Walk around to the opposite side of your subject and scan in from that side. See if you can detect the overall shape and strength of the energy aura. Is it uniform? Does it feel 7 inches deep all the way around? Or, does one side feel 3 inches deep while another feels 9 inches deep? Does it feel relatively strong or weak?

9. Conclude the exercise by walking around for a few minutes and shaking your arms and legs. Relax and take a few deep breaths.

After you've finished, you may want to jot down your scanning impressions of your subject's aura so that you can refer to them later.

If you are able to practice on different subjects, try to get a sense of the relative strength of people's auras. Jot down these scanning impressions for comparison with your other efforts.

As you perform general scanning on different people, you'll be surprised at how quickly you pick up the ability—and how accurate it can be. A fourteen-year-old student in Minnesota, J. D. Thomas, helped out at a Pranic Healing clinic the day after completing his first class. As he scanned a woman, he felt some energetic disturbances in her lower abdomen and lower back and got an impression that she might have a bladder problem, perhaps an infection. He mentioned this to the woman, and she confirmed that she was having trouble with her bladder. He then applied the appropriate healing technique (similar to the energetic remedies in Chapter 13), and the woman left the clinic feeling much better.

SCANNING CHECKLIST

1. Place your tongue on your palate.
2. Perform a few cycles of pranic breathing.

3. Tap your heart chakra several times with any two fingers of your scanning hand.

4. At minimum, do Hand Sensitivity Exercise 1. You can do Hand Sensitivity Exercise 2 if you have the time or just want to increase your sensitivity even more.

5. Keep your fingers, hand, wrist, and arm relaxed; keep your armpit open.

6. Look briefly at your scanning target to establish your intent to scan.

7. Breathe slowly and deeply as you scan.

8. Keep your awareness on the palm chakra of the scanning hand. Look at your target first, but as you scan keep your awareness on the palm chakra of the scanning hand. Your concentration level should be about the same level you use in reading a book. Remember, in scanning, you are feeling the flow of energy rather than seeing it. Keeping your awareness on the scanning hand emphasizes feeling rather than seeing the energy.

9. Keep your eyes open or closed, whichever helps you to sustain your focus better.

10. Keep a positive, open-minded attitude. Doubts, fears, and apprehensions inhibit your ability to sense subtle energy.

SIX STEPS DAILY PRACTICE ROUTINE—UPDATE

1. *Direct clearing* (Exercises 3–A and 3–B). As needed.

2. *Stretching and loosening the diaphragm* (Exercise 4–A). Once your diaphragm is opened up, you may want to perform these exercises only occasionally, just to add variety to your routine.

3. *Hand Sensitivity Exercises 1 and 2* (Exercises 1–A and 5–A).

4. *Pranic breathing* (Exercise 4–B). Do three sets of ten pranic breaths. Progress to the 7–1–7–1 and then 6–3–6–3 rhythm and retention sequences.

5. *General scanning* (Exercises 5–B and 5–E). Practice on a variety of targets: your arm, your leg, and other parts of your body; plants, animals, other people.

As you move into practicing hands-on energy manipulation—scanning in this chapter and the next, and sweeping and energizing in the following chapters—remember to try to build a good foundation of sensitivity as you take your practice step by step. But if you're not feeling the energy at a particular step after a while, just move on to the next exercise. Some people take a little longer than others.

In the next chapter, you'll learn specific or targeted scanning.

CHAPTER 6

Hands Up!
More Scanning—
Specific Scanning and
Interpreting Results

"A man brought his eighteen-month-old daughter, who was suffering from chronic kidney infections, into our clinic. The doctors could find no reason for the recurring infections, but they knew the left kidney was shrinking and dying. A nephrologist had told the father that unless they could find a way to stop the infections, the infant would need a kidney transplant. I performed general scanning on her aura, and then specific scanning on her chakras and lower back. The energy in her right kidney felt strong and normal, but I got no feeling of energy at all in the left kidney. We began Pranic Healing treatments. I swept and energized the kidneys and the related chakras—the ajna, the basic, the sex, and the meng mein. After about a year of weekly and then twice-weekly treatments, the infections stopped, her condition stabilized, and she was able to go off all antibiotics. Their doctor was baffled by the child's improvement. Moreover, the doctor said that, over that year of treatment with Pranic Healing, the left kidney had grown larger than the right one. Nearly three years later, the little girl is now perfectly normal and healthy."

—KIM FANTINI, BELLEVILLE, ILLINOIS

In these next exercises, we'll discuss targeted or *specific scanning*, which is feeling the prana at particular points or areas in your energetic anatomy. Specific scanning includes feeling the energy of both individual chakras and body parts, but in the exercises here you'll use the chakras only as scanning targets because they're better targets for beginners. Once you can scan chakras successfully, you can easily scan particular parts of the body. In this chapter, you'll also learn what the energy sensations you get from scanning actually mean.

In general scanning, you scanned the aura for two characteristics: depth and strength. You scan chakras for three characteristics: depth, strength, and *width*. Chakras can be deep and strong but narrow, or shallow and weak but wide. You scan chakras for width in order to get a complete picture of their energy.

SPECIFIC SELF-SCANNING

As you begin more targeted or specific self-scanning, make sure you keep your intent clear and firm to ensure accuracy. Beginning Pranic Healing students can misread their aura without clear intent. Says Pranic Healing student Naila Vavra, "When I first began scanning, my biggest concern was that I would confuse one chakra for another or get a reading on the size of the aura instead of a specific chakra. 'Intent' was the magic word. The moment my intent was focused and I would silently say to myself, for example, 'width of heart chakra,' I would get an accurate reading instantly. When the intent is clear, the reading is accurate, and I can trust it."

EXERCISE 6–A: *Specific Self-Scanning—Scanning Chakras for Depth and Strength*

Located in the soft area just below the sternum or breastbone, the front solar plexus chakra (Figure 6–1) is a clearinghouse or way station for prana moving back and forth between the upper and lower chakras. As you read in Chapter 1, it is also the seat of the lower emotions, and as such, it's a particularly good chakra to scan to get a quick sense of your overall well-being.

You may sit or stand during this exercise. Perform your four-step warm-up, then proceed.

FIGURE 6–1

1. Begin with your scanning hand about 2 to 3 feet out in front of your body, not quite at full arm's length. Your palm should face back toward your body.

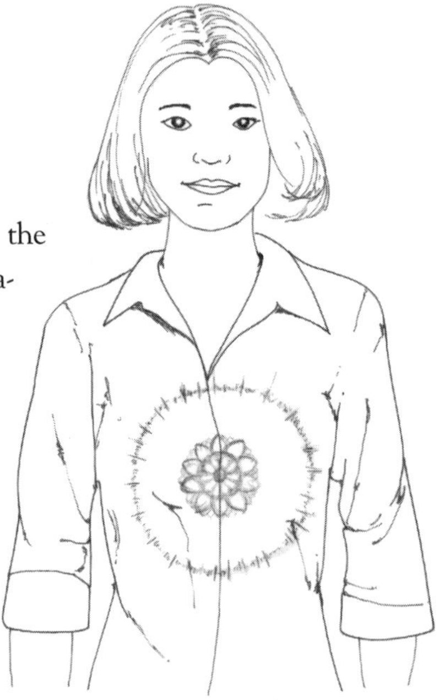

2. Look down at your target to tune in and form your intent to scan.

3. Breathe slowly and deeply, using pranic breathing. Once you have looked at the front solar plexus to establish your intent, keep your awareness on your scanning hand throughout the rest of the exercise. Keep a positive, open-minded attitude.

4. Move your scanning hand slowly toward your front solar plexus chakra, keeping your hand open and relaxed, your palm facing your body, and your wrist loose. Keep your fingers in a natural, relaxed position— slightly curved and open (Figure 6–2). Slow down even more as your palm gets about a foot away from your body.

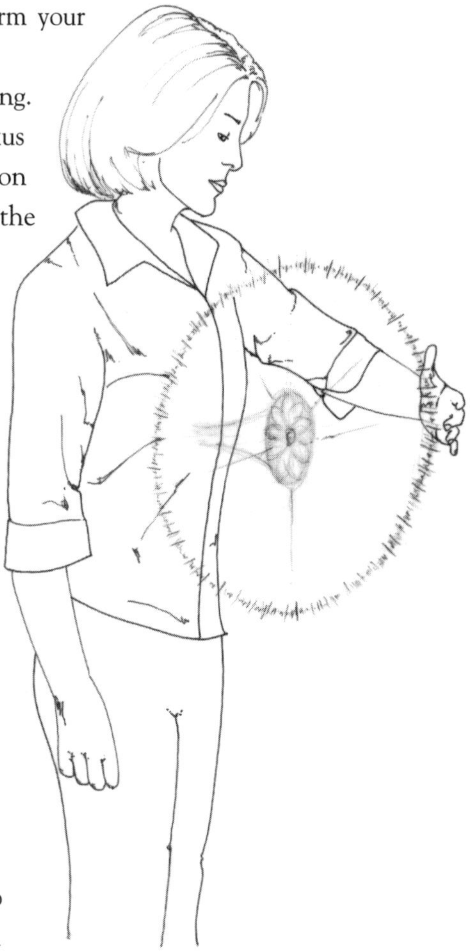

5. Now move your scanning hand forward and back in front of your solar plexus chakra several times gently, breathing slowly and deeply. Your hand should move within a range of 4 to 12 inches in front of your solar plexus chakra, neither touching nor moving more than a foot away from your body. Try to feel the energy of your front solar plexus with your scanning hand as it moves in toward your body and out again. Keep your arm joints loose and supple as you move your scanning hand forward and back.

FIGURE 6–2

6. Stop your hand when you get that feeling of pressure, tingling, or heat in your palm. You should feel this sensation as you get within 4 to 6 inches of your body. The inner aura of the average healthy adult, which includes the aura of the chakras, is about 5 inches in depth. But chakras have a more concentrated feeling than the general aura, so you should feel a stronger impression of energy as you scan the front solar plexus chakra than when you scanned your arm.

7. As in the other exercises, if you don't feel the energy right away, don't be discouraged. Relax, breathe deeply, and move your hand back from your body and then in again

until you feel it. If after 5 minutes you still have difficulty feeling the energy, take a few minutes and repeat Hand Sensitivity Exercise 1 or 2. Or practice with plants, animals, and other people a bit more before scanning your own chakras.

8. Also, as in previous exercises, when you feel the pressure, tingling, or warmth in your hand, notice how far away your hand is from your body. Is it that average of 5 inches away? Is it closer or farther? Note the depth. Don't worry for now if it's deeper or shallower than 5 inches.

9. As you scan for depth, get a sense of the *strength* of the chakra as well. Ask yourself the same questions you did in the previous scanning exercises: Do you feel a strong sense of pressure or tingling? Does it feel like your hand is being repelled forcefully? Or do you feel only slight pressure? Continue scanning until you get a feel for the depth and strength of your front solar plexus chakra.

10. Conclude the exercise by walking around for a few minutes and shaking your arms and legs. Relax and take a few deep breaths.

After you've finished, you may want to jot down your scanning impressions so that you can refer to them later.

If you don't strongly feel the energy in this exercise, you may wonder if you have an underpowered front solar plexus chakra. This is possible, but it's more likely that you haven't developed sufficient sensitivity to feel the energy. Just keep an open attitude and stick with your practice; you'll develop the ability to feel the energy.

EXERCISE 6–B: *Specific Self-Scanning—Scanning Chakras for Width*

To scan for width, you use *both* hands. Since you scan for width right after scanning for depth and strength, you needn't perform the warm-up again, even if you've taken a break for a few minutes. If you feel you're getting mentally fatigued or need to recharge your sensitivity, though, tap your heart again and take a few pranic breaths before proceeding.

1. Extend your arms waist-high, in the holding-a-beach-ball position. Your hands should be about 3 feet apart, elbows at a 90-degree angle, palms directly facing each other and forearms parallel to the ground.

2. To scan the width of your front solar plexus chakra, you have to raise your hands slightly from your initial waist-high position and place them at the same level as your front solar plexus chakra. Then pull them straight back toward your body. As you do this, however,

remember to keep your hands 3 feet apart and keep your palms facing each other. It will be as if you're lifting the beach ball and pulling it straight back toward you. This is your starting posture (Figure 6–3).

3. Tune in to your target and form your intent to scan.

4. Scan in slowly with both hands. Take your time. Breathe deeply. Your scanning motion is the slow-motion clapping used in the Hand Sensitivity Exercises. As your wrists approach your ribs, your hands will be about 10 inches apart. Slow down even more. When your open palms are about 6 to 8 inches apart, they will be approaching the sides of the front solar plexus chakra. At this point, begin to feel for the perimeter of the front solar plexus chakra, with that in-and-out slow-motion clapping.

5. Stop when you feel that tingling, resistance, pressure, or warmth. It should be a stronger

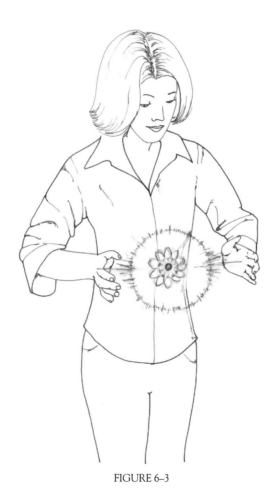

FIGURE 6–3

or more concentrated feeling than what you felt in scanning your aura. Try to determine the diameter of the front solar plexus chakra. A healthy adult will have a front solar plexus chakra about 4 inches in diameter. If yours appears to be narrower or wider than 4 inches, don't be concerned now. Simply note the width.

6. If you don't feel any resistance or heat as you approach the sides of the front solar plexus chakra, don't be discouraged. Do a few more cycles of pranic breathing; perform Hand Sensitivity Exercise 1 or 2. Or, if you are completely unable to feel the energy, go back to a previous step in the progressive exercise sequence at which you were able to feel the energy—such as the hand sensitivity exercises, scanning your arm, scanning a plant— and then build up to scanning the width of the chakras.

7. Conclude the exercise by walking around for a few minutes and shaking your arms and legs. Relax and take a few deep breaths. Jot down your scanning impressions.

Scanning the Other Front Chakras

Using the same steps described in Exercises 6–A and 6–B, now scan the other chakras on the front of your body. Refer to Figure 1–1 and Table 1–I for these locations.

Shake your hands and fingers, and reestablish your intent before scanning each of these chakras. Scan them for depth, strength, and width. Compare their relative depth, strength, and width. After you finish scanning each chakra, you may wish to write down the measurements and any other impressions you develop.

If at any time you feel mentally fatigued or feel you're losing your concentration or sensitivity, stop and take a break. Perform a few cycles of pranic breathing. Walk around, or repeat your four-step warm-up sequence.

After you have finished scanning your front chakras, you may move on to scan your back chakras.

SCANNING USING VISUALIZATION

Scanning Your Back Chakras Using Visualization

Obviously, it's impossible to reach around your back with your hand to scan your back chakras, so you scan them with visualization. You conceive a mental picture of yourself out in front of you and then scan the back chakras of that visualization. Refer to Figure 1–1 and Table 1–I for the location of your back chakras.

Visualization Tips

There are different ways to visualize yourself, and no one method works best for everyone, but here are some tips and considerations. Experiment to find out which visualization style works best for you.

- Many find it helpful to close their eyes before starting to visualize, while others keep their eyes open but unfocused, gazing at nothing in particular, as if they were daydreaming.
- If you're literal-minded, try seeing a life-size representation of yourself about 2 or 3 feet directly in front of you. You can visualize it against a blank screen. Some people like to see a black screen; others find that a white screen, similar to a movie theater screen, works better. Still others like to visualize the image right in front of them in the room; they like the 3-D quality of such a visualization.
- Some people like details. If well-defined pictures help you, make your visualization as anatomically correct as you can. You may even want to consult a medical text for reference. Add colors and depth perception. Other people like a simpler two-dimensional cartoonlike or animated representation.
- Imagine drawing yourself on a white board with markers or painting on a canvas with vivid colors.
- Some people like to work in life-size images; others prefer a less-than-full-size representation, half-size or smaller, and feel they can concentrate better on a smaller image. In Pranic Healing classes, students are taught to scan a visualization of themselves that is one-half or one-third their normal size or even smaller, a technique that most find very helpful. "I scanned myself using this method and was amazed that I could actually feel pranic congestion as a bump in the solar plexus," says Tracy Johns. "I've also used this for distant scanning (scanning someone who is not in the room with you)."
- Creative people with more developed visualization skills may try the microscope technique, in which they blow up or zoom in on a particular chakra or area of a possible health problem.
- Try visualization to scan your front chakras. Once you have learned to scan a visualization of your back chakras, you may find that you prefer to use a visualization rather than your physical body to scan your front chakras as well. This is fine.

EXERCISE 6–C: *Scanning Your Back Chakras*

You may sit or stand during this exercise. Perform your four-step warm-up, then proceed.

1. Use your preferred visualization method to project an image of yourself out in front of you. Turn it around so that you are facing the back of your image.

2. Locate your back solar plexus chakra (Figure 6–4). Tune in to your target and form your intent to scan. Here is another way to increase your sensitivity when scanning a visualization: Repeat your name three times before beginning—for instance, "John Smith, John Smith, John Smith." This is a simple but extremely powerful technique for increasing sensitivity. At this point in class, students first scan the back of their aura for congestion or depletion without any special instructions. Then they are instructed to say their own name three times before scanning, then repeat the scanning exercise. Invari-

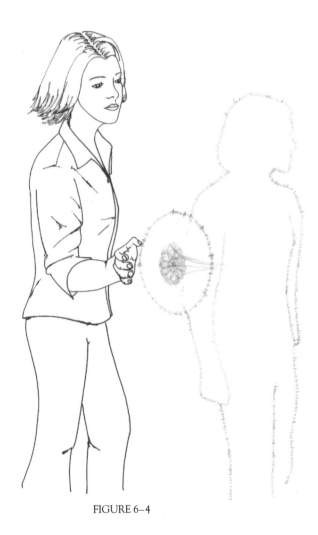

FIGURE 6–4

ably, the students find that all tactile sensations—pressure, temperature, tingling—are much more distinct.

3. Breathe slowly and deeply, using pranic breathing. Once you have looked at your target chakra to establish your intent, keep your awareness on your scanning hand throughout the rest of the scanning exercise. Keep a positive, open-minded attitude.

4. Raise your scanning hand, and with your palm open and your wrist loose, begin scanning by moving your hand toward your targeted spot. Scan your back solar plexus chakra in the same way you scanned your front solar plexus chakra, feeling for its depth, strength, and width.

5. It requires more concentration to scan a visualization, so go slowly, breathe deeply, and keep your awareness on the palm chakra of your scanning hand.

6. When you're finished scanning your back solar plexus chakra for depth, strength, and width, take a moment and jot down your impressions. Then either move to scanning the next back chakra or, if you need to take a break, take a few deep breaths and walk around for a minute or two.

INTERPRETING YOUR SCANNING RESULTS

The interpretation of your scanning results is a two-part process. First, you establish your *energetic baseline*, the general size and strength of your entire aura at a particular time, which provides a general indication of your overall energy level and well-being. Next, you establish your *chakral baseline*, the size and strength of individual chakras, which gives you a sense of some specific indicators of your health and well-being.

Your Energetic Baseline

In Chapter 5, you scanned the inside of your forearm and several other parts of your body to get a rough idea of the general strength of your aura. But no single measurement by itself provides an accurate assessment of your aura's overall size and strength. To get this overall reading, you need to scan your entire energetic anatomy. But you don't have to scan yourself at dozens of points from head to toe. There's a better, quicker way.

For your baseline, divide your body into four quadrants—low, middle, high, and top—and perform a specific scanning routine on two key points in each of the four quadrants: the outside of both knees (low quadrant), the outside of both hips (middle quadrant), the inside of both forearms (high quadrant), and both temples (top quadrant). These particular points are easy to reach, and taken together, they yield a representative reading of your entire aura. This shortcut enables you to establish your energetic baseline in minutes.

You scan these eight points in the four quadrants three times in a row in the same order: knees, hips, forearms, and then temples. This is one set. Then scan them a second time in the same order; that's the second set. Finally, scan them a third time, which is your third set.

Scanning a target several times in a row until the same readings are produced each time is the best way to ensure accuracy. For beginners especially, consistent results mean accurate results. When you become proficient, you will be able to scan once and interpret accurately and confidently. But we've seen in class that when beginning scanners try to interpret before they produce consistent readings, their results are unpredictable, incomplete, or erroneous. As a result, they become frustrated and begin to question whether scanning and this "energy stuff" really work.

As a beginner, you get more accurate readings and learn more quickly by scanning in sets instead of scanning the knee three times in a row, then the hip three times in a row, and so on, because you break contact with the scanning target between scans. If you don't break contact between scans, you may be unconsciously influenced by your first scan. You may remember, for instance, that on your first scan of the hip, your hand stopped at 5 inches deep, so that when you follow up right away with a second scan of the hip, you may think that it should stop at 5 inches deep as well. Perhaps it should; perhaps that first scan was correct. But with beginners who haven't fully developed their scanning ability, it's also quite possible that the first scan wasn't accurate. Scanning in sets ensures accuracy.

EXERCISE 6–D: *Establishing Your Energetic Baseline*

You may sit or stand during this exercise. Perform your four-step warm-up, then proceed.

1. Scan the outside of your right knee with your right hand, noting the depth and strength of the aura. Scan the outside of your left knee with your left hand, noting the depth and strength of the aura. If you wish, you can scan both knees at the same time with both hands.
2. Scan your right hip with your right hand, noting the depth and strength of the aura. Scan your left hip with your left hand, noting the depth and strength of the aura. As above, if you wish, you can scan both hips at the same time with both hands.

3. Scan your forearm as you did in Exercise 5–B in the last chapter; then reverse your hands and scan your other forearm.

4. Scan your head at your right temple with your right hand, noting the depth and strength of the aura. Scan your head at your left temple with your left hand, noting the depth and strength of the aura. As with the above steps, if you wish, you can scan both temples at the same time with both hands.

5. Take a break for a minute or two.

6. Repeat this sequence until you get the same depth and strength measurements from two or three consecutive sets of scanning.

When you get consistent results from those four points—for example, after three sets of scanning, you've determined that your aura is 5 inches deep at each point all the way around; or, it's 3 inches deep at the right knee, 6 at the right hip, 4 at both temples, etc.—this measurement is your energetic baseline.

Here is what this measurement means: If your aura is uniformly large—for example, 10 inches deep at all eight points—it's likely that you are very healthy and highly energized. If your aura is uniformly small—for example, 2 inches deep at all eight points—this indicates a general condition of low energy, which may manifest as any number of health problems. If your aura is irregular in size—for example, your aura extends out 8 inches at the right hip and 3 inches at the left temple—you have an energetic imbalance. In an irregular aura, a larger-than-average area is evidence of local congestion, while a smaller-than-average area indicates local depletion. Energetic congestion is a thickened protrusion of dirty energy and is felt differently by different people. Our students describe it as a "bulge"; it feels like the repelling force you get when bringing the north poles of two magnets together. Energetic depletion is a gap in the aura that is almost always felt during scanning as a depression in the energy field. Your hand actually sinks in toward the body as it passes over the area. Congestion or depletion may indicate a present or imminent health problem in the area where you have an imbalance. In upcoming chapters you will learn how to clear away or *sweep* local congestion, as well as how to *energize* local areas of depletion.

A word of caution: You may be able to infer a particular health problem from your own scanning and from Table 1–I, which associates the chakras with certain organs or body functions. Do not attempt to diagnose yourself or anyone else! Take the information to a doctor you trust for further diagnosis and treatment. In this book, you are learning a program that has been demonstrated to be effective in addressing certain medical conditions that already exist and have been diagnosed. We do not encourage readers to diagnose themselves on the basis of scanning the energetic anatomy. *Your Hands Can Heal You*, Pranic

Healing, and energy medicine in general are powerful tools that are meant to complement, not replace, traditional Western medicine.

Energetic Baseline Variations

The size of your aura varies throughout the day and night, as your energy level is affected by many factors, including the food you eat, your emotional state, the amount of stress you're under, and so on. If you've found your aura varying between 4 and 6 inches deep over the course of several days, these modulations are normal. More dramatic changes—for instance, you find your aura shrinking to 2 inches overall, or you find bulges out to 9 inches in some areas—are the types of energetic disturbances that could be indicators of health problems.

Your Chakral Baseline

The most complete picture of specific energetic indicators of health comes from scanning all eleven major chakras to determine the size and strength of each. As you did in establishing your general energetic baseline, you scan your chakras sequentially in several sets in order to ensure consistent, accurate readings. Once you become a more proficient scanner, you can scan for the depth, strength, and width of your chakras in a single set. The direction and sequence in which you scan your chakras does not affect the quality of your readings. But, so that you have some order and structure in the early stages of your practice, this sequence is recommended: crown, forehead, *ajna*, throat, front heart, front solar plexus, front spleen, navel, sex, basic, *meng mein*, back spleen, back solar plexus, and back heart.

EXERCISE 6–E: *Establishing Your Chakral Baseline*

You may sit or stand during this exercise. Perform your four-step warm-up, then proceed.

1. Scan your 11 major chakras for all three dimensions as you learned to do in Exercises 6–A, 6–B, and 6–C. Remember to use your intent to focus on the chakra rather than the general aura and also to sense for that feeling of concentration that differentiates a chakra from the aura. Note the depth, strength, and width of each chakra.
2. Take a break for a few minutes.
3. Repeat this sequence—scanning the major chakras in the order presented above, then taking a break—until you get consistent readings two or three times in a row.
   When you get consistent readings, you can interpret your results. Interpretation of your

chakral baseline is similar to interpretating your energetic baseline. The chakras of the average healthy adult are about 5 inches deep and 4 inches wide. If all your chakras are larger than average, it's likely that you are healthy and highly energized. If all your chakras are smaller than average, it's likely that you have a general condition of low energy, which may manifest as any number of health problems. If your chakras vary in size—for example, if they have different widths and depths, and some feel substantially stronger or weaker than others—then you have an imbalance in your energetic body that may indicate a present or imminent health problem. A larger-than-average chakra is evidence of congestion; a smaller-than-average chakra indicates depletion. If there is an energetic disturbance in a particular chakra, a health problem may result in the organ or bodily function controlled by that chakra. For example, if your navel and basic chakras are depleted, this may manifest as a state of general low energy or as an ailment that causes reduced overall energy. If your *meng mein* chakra is congested or overactivated, this may show up as high blood pressure. In the chapters ahead, you will learn how to sweep away congestion and energize areas of depletion.

Chakra Baseline Variations

The size of your chakras, like the size of your general aura, is constantly expanding and contracting within a range that enables you to determine whether a particular chakra is unusually large or small, strong or weak, and thus a possible indicator of a specific health problem. A healthy chakra does not vary in size and strength suddenly and dramatically, but as with the general aura, it will have subtle variations throughout the day and night.

SIX STEPS DAILY PRACTICE ROUTINE—UPDATE

1. *Direct clearing* (Exercises 4–A and 4B). As needed.
2. *Stretching and loosening the diaphragm* (Exercise 4–A). As needed, or for variety.
3. *Hand Sensitivity Exercise 1 or 2* (Exercise 1–A or 5–A).
4. *Pranic breathing* (Exercise 4–B). Use your preferred rhythm and retention.
5. *General scanning* (Exercises 5–B to 5–E). Practice on a variety of targets: your arm, your leg, and other parts of your body; plants, animals, other people. Add: energetic baseline (Exercise 6–D).
6. *Specific scanning.* Practice on small targets (for example, your left wrist or right ear), individual chakras (Exercises 6–A and 6–B), chakral baseline (Exercise 6–E), self-scanning using visualization (Exercise 6–C), specific scanning with your nondominant hand.

As you learn more techniques, you may not have time to practice them all every day. This is fine. You may wish to practice some on different days, or to create several routines for variety. You'll also be able to save a little time as you become a better scanner. For instance, you may not need to practice the hand sensitivity exercises regularly, because your sensitivity will be well-developed. All you'll need to do is place your tongue on the roof of your mouth, perform a few cycles of pranic breathing, do a quick hand sensitivity exercise (either 1 or 2), and tap your heart chakra, and you'll be ready to scan.

In the next chapter, you'll learn the second of the energy-manipulation techniques, sweeping.

CHAPTER 7

Out With the Old— Sweeping Away Congested Energy, Cleaning Your Aura

"I often work very long days on hard concrete stage floors. This can be very hard on the body. After about six hours, the pain begins in my feet and works its way up to my legs, knees, and lower back. It also becomes difficult to concentrate late in the day (which is when my job is most challenging). I used to take aspirin and coffee to get me through the day, but that made my stomach a mess and made me cranky. I've found general and localized sweeping to be a simple miracle. I sweep 'tired' away from my eyes, the pain from my feet, knees, and lower back, and I can continue my work with surprising energy and a smile. It's made me a better director, and I am forever grateful. Thank you! Sweeping takes a few moments, and the relief lasts for hours."

—PAM D., LOS ANGELES

Cleanliness is a vital part of every healing approach. Traditional medicine seeks to minimize dirt and germs that cause infection. That's why a nurse swabs an open cut with peroxide, and a surgeon thoroughly scrubs his hands and arms before operating. Nontraditional energy medicine, too, is concerned with cleanliness: It seeks to remove energetic contamination from the aura that could lead to health problems. In India certain healers wave a peacock feather over the body, and in the Philippines, healers brush the patient with a special broom. All these modalities are quite different, but the philosophy behind them is the same: In order to be healthy, the body must be clean of impurities, whether they are microbes or dirty prana.

In this chapter, you will learn *sweeping*, the Pranic Healing method of ensuring energetic cleanliness by manually removing contamination, or dirty energy, from your aura. Sweeping is the second of the three energy manipulation techniques.

THE BASICS OF SWEEPING

There are two types of sweeping, general sweeping and local sweeping. *General sweeping* is a series of 10 two-handed sweeps—five down the front of the body and five down the back—that constitutes an overall head-to-toe and front-to-back cleansing of the energetic anatomy. *Local sweeping* is more targeted manual cleansing of a specific body part or chakra. Local sweeping is carried out with one hand, and the cleansing is deeper and more concentrated.

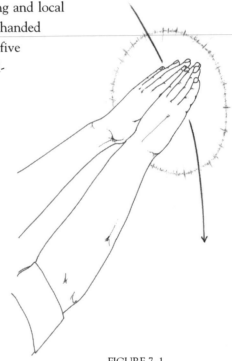

To perform general sweeping, you use both hands in long, slow, graceful, hands-cupped movements (Figure 7–1). This induces what is called the *healing state*, a condition of advanced physical and mental relaxation in which you are optimally receptive to healing energy—and to healing. People describe this super-relaxed state as "a tremendous release of tension," "all the heaviness is gone," or "a feeling of lightness." This relaxation is due to removal of dirty

FIGURE 7–1

prana from the energy body and indirect clearing of negative emotions. As you sweep away the energetic blockages or functional boundaries from your aura, your body and mind fully relax.

Here's another way to look at the healing state. Electrical current passes easily through high-grade wire because the metal from which the wire is fashioned has few impurities. By contrast, electricity passes through low-grade wire with more difficulty because the metal from which low-grade wire is created has many impurities. A clean energy body in the healing state is like high-grade wire; prana flows through it smoothly. A dirty energy body is like low-grade wire; prana can't flow through it very well because it's full of impurities, or ener-

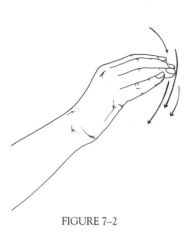

FIGURE 7–2

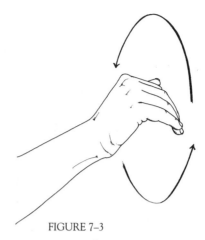

FIGURE 7–3

getic congestion. As prana tries to move through a dirty aura, it clogs up even more, leading to greater energetic imbalances and eventually health problems.

Local sweeping employs two hand motions, a dog paddle–type motion (Figure 7–2) and a tight counterclockwise twisting motion (Figure 7–3), to provide more focused cleansing of smaller areas of your energy body. When you perform local sweeping on yourself with the counterclockwise twisting motion, your orientation for determining counterclockwise is always from outside your body looking back at it. If you ever get confused, simply imagine—or even *place*—a clock facing outward on the body part on which you're working and follow the hands of the clock (Figure 7–4). When you perform local sweeping on a visualization of yourself, as you will later on, the same rule applies. Imagine a clock on the part of the visualization on which you are working, and follow the hands of the clock.

There are also several ways to use your hand in local sweeping: with the fingers pointed toward your target (for penetrating cleansing); with the inside or outside edge of the hand (for softer cleansing, and to clean areas that are awkward to reach with a fingers-pointed hand posture); and with one or two fingers (in a poking motion to loosen up tough areas of congestion).

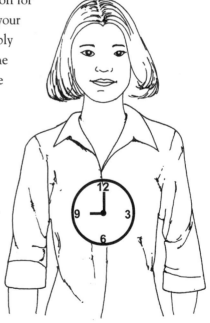

FIGURE 7–4

ADDITIONAL SAFEGUARDS FOR HIGHER-LEVEL ENERGY MANIPULATION

With sweeping, you begin higher-level energy manipulation, and you must take further steps to protect yourself against contamination. These steps will be even more important when you begin energizing (Chapter 8) and practicing remedies for specific ailments (Chapter 13). Please add the following steps to your practice from this point forward.

1. *Before you begin, remove clothing and items that can pick up dirty energy.* Roll up your sleeves, take off your shoes and belt, and empty your pockets of money, keys, and other items. The long sleeves of shirts, especially cotton, get contaminated easily, and silk is an insulator that prevents the flow of energy. Leather is also an insulator. Since money passes through so many hands, it tends to be very dirty energetically and can contaminate your healing energy.

2. *Dispose of dirty energy properly.* The simplest and most effective way to neutralize the dirty energy that you sweep away from your aura is to throw it into a nearby bowl of salt water (Figure 7–5). As you'll read in Chapter 10, salt neutralizes dirty energy. To prepare your saline "disposal unit," take a bowl or plastic container that holds about a quart, fill it two-thirds with water, and then pour in about 6 to 8 ounces of salt. You can use either table salt or rock salt, the kind that is used to melt ice and snow on roads (but not Epsom salts; they don't have the same energetic cleansing ability). When you're finished with each sweeping/healing session, throw the dirty salt water into the toilet and flush it. If no salt water is available, visualize that you have a green fire burning in a bucket at your side, and throw the dirty energy into it. When you are finished sweeping, extinguish the flame by visualizing a bucket of water pouring on it.

3. *Keep your sweeping/energizing arm clean.* As you

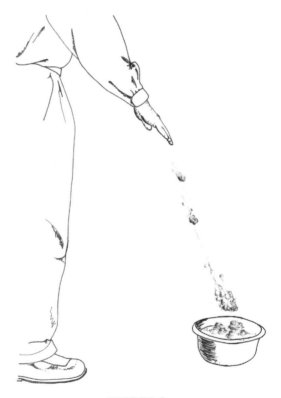

FIGURE 7–5

sweep, you will find that your hand and arm may feel heavy. This is partly due to the repetitive physical motion of sweeping, but more due to your arm picking up dirty energy. Keep your sweeping hand and arm from becoming unnecessarily contaminated by spraying them every ten sweeps with alcohol, witch hazel, or salt water. A mister used to spray houseplants is perfect. If the nozzle is adjustable, set it to its finest spray. You can also use a small pump sprayer, which you can find at your local drugstore. As you become more proficient and more able to detect just how contaminated your hands are getting, you can spray as necessary, but in the beginning, just spray every ten total sweeps. (*Note:* From this point forward, when we make references to "alcohol" or an "alcohol bottle," understand that you could also have witch hazel or salt water in your "alcohol bottle.")

4. *Begin practice/healing session by invoking.* As you work with more energy that comes from outside your body, you may need some guidance in your healing work. Thus before starting any self-healing routine, we suggest that you invoke a higher being, saint, or deity of your choice. It helps ensure safe practice and the safety of anyone on whom you may practice. You can use a favorite prayer or inspirational passage, or even direct your invocation to an undefined higher power. It can be simple and brief. Here's an example: "Thank you, _____, for this healing energy and for the guidance to use it safely and properly."

5. *If you work with a woman who is or may be pregnant, you should practice only scanning and mild sweeping.* Strong sweeping, energizing, and colored pranas can damage a fetus. There are sweeping and energizing routines for pregnant women, but they are reserved for experienced pranic healers. You'll see additional warnings on working with pregnant women in the chapters on energizing (Chapter 8) and using colored pranas (Chapter 9).

6. *End a session in which you practice on someone else by cutting cords.* Any time you work energetically with someone else, especially if the person has a health problem or energetic disturbance, you establish an "energetic rapport" that takes the form of a pranic thread or cord between your energy body and theirs. If you leave this cord intact when you're finished, dirty energy can flow back to you through the cord and contaminate you. For instance, one instructor had been performing Pranic Healing on her father for a bone spur on his foot. After several sessions over two weeks, her father reported his condition much improved, but the instructor's foot began to hurt, and she couldn't figure out why. When she remembered that she hadn't cut the cord between her father and herself, she did so, and her foot pain went away.

Cutting the cord prevents contamination. At the end of your session, simply visualize a thread between you and your subject. See your hand as a knife and cut the cord close to your front solar plexus with a brisk karate chop–like motion.

PROGRESSIVE SWEEPING EXERCISES

Here is the sequence of progressive sweeping exercises:

1. Presweeping hand preparation
2. General sweeping of another person
3. General sweeping of the health rays of another person
4. Local sweeping of another person
5. General self-sweeping
6. General self-sweeping of your health rays
7. Local self-sweeping

Note that you will practice sweeping on other people before you begin self-sweeping. We have found in classes that it is generally easier for students to learn sweeping (and energizing, too) by beginning on someone else first. As with scanning, we are presenting an *optimal* sequence for learning to sweep. Just as you can still learn scanning if you don't have plants and animals on which to practice by practicing more on yourself, you can still learn sweeping if you don't have a practice partner. You simply work more on the self-sweeping exercises. Do your best to follow this sequence, but if you can't, you can still learn to scan through consistent, regular practice of the steps you can practice.

Most people pick up sweeping within a couple weeks of daily practice after developing reasonably good hand sensitivity and scanning ability. But, as with scanning, if you get stuck at one step, just move on to the next exercise. You'll pick it up before too long.

PRESWEEPING HAND PREPARATION

The presweeping hand preparation sequence is essentially advanced hand sensitivity. It's also like hand sensitivity in that you learn it first as a stand-alone exercise, then as you progress, integrate it into your normal self-healing routine.

EXERCISE 7–A: *Presweeping Hand Preparation*

You may sit or stand for this exercise. Perform your four-step warm-up, then proceed.

Sweeping Heals!

"The Tibetan master Djwhal Khul said, 'All disease is a result of inhibited Soul Life. . . . The art of the healer consists of releasing the Soul, so that it can flow through the aggregate of organisms which constitute any particular form. . . . The true and future healing is brought about when the life of the Soul can flow without impediment and hindrance throughout every aspect of the form. It can then vitalize it.' What this means is, the more abundantly spiritual energy (Soul Life) flows into the body through the crown chakra, the faster will be the rate of healing. This is where sweeping comes in. By properly sweeping and removing the blockages in the energy aura, the Soul Life can flow in easily through the crown and then go on to various parts of the body.

"The use of purposeful sweeping distinguishes Pranic Healing from other energy medicine modalities. Instead of simply giving energy to a sick person, pranic healers perform extensive sweeping first to remove energetic blockages that might hinder the intake of the purest healing energy of all, divine energy, or Soul Life. In fact, as you will read later on, the optimum ratio of sweeping to energizing in Pranic Healing is four or five to one."

—*Master Stephen Co*

1. From the basic hand sensitivity exercise position, with elbows at 90 degrees, turn your palms upward.
2. Move your upper arms slightly away from the body to open up the armpits a little more.
3. Invoke to offer thanks for the healing energy, the knowledge to use it properly, and safety in using it.
4. Place your awareness on the palm chakras of both hands and perform three cycles of pranic breathing. You may feel your hands become warm, flushed, or tingly, and this is perfectly fine.

You're now ready to sweep.

GENERAL SWEEPING OF ANOTHER PERSON

The principal benefit of practicing sweeping on another person is feedback. When students begin sweeping, they're often unsure if they're performing the technique properly and if they're producing results. Thus, immediate comments from a subject are invaluable to developing confidence in higher-level energy manipulation. You can ask your subject before you sweep if she has any current health problems and then after sweeping, if she feels any different.

EXERCISE 7–B: *General Sweeping of Another Person*

Stand for this exercise. Perform your standard four-step warm-up, and then add the following four steps as well. (From this point forward, include the first two of the following steps in your warm-up before all practice sessions that include sweeping or energizing. Add all four steps if you're working on another person.)

- Have your bowl of salt water and sprayer filled with either alcohol, witch hazel, or salt water handy. Keep the bowl of salt water within several feet but off to the side so you won't trip over it.
- Perform Presweeping Hand Preparation (Exercise 7–A), including invocation.
- Ask your subject if he has any current health problems. (You may or may not want him to divulge them. If he tells you what they are, that may predispose you to remember where they are, and the learning experience of the exercise may be less powerful. If he does not tell you and you uncover an energetic disturbance associated with them, it's a huge confidence-booster. But you may want the help in the beginning. Experiment and see which way helps you learn better.)
- Tell your subject to keep his tongue on the roof of his mouth to increase sensitivity.

1. Scan your subject at several points to establish a quick energetic baseline. In establishing your own energetic baseline, you scanned four quadrants in three sets. Here you don't need that level of detail. You just want a rough sense of the depth and strength of your subject's aura at a couple of points. Scan the left and then the right shoulder several times until you get a feel for the basic strength and contour of your subject's energetic anatomy. Even if you can't feel the energy perfectly, just proceed with the sweeping exercise. Sweeping increases your sensitivity, too.
2. Reestablish your intent by silently declaring to yourself that you intend to sweep and clean away the dirty prana from this person's energy body.
3. With your hands in the slightly cupped general sweeping position, bring your hands together so that the forefingers and inside edge of the hands touch (Photo 7–a), and aim your fingers slightly above your subject's head. If you are standing about 3 feet away, your hands will be about 4 to 6 inches from your subject's body. As you progress,

you'll find that you can scan and sweep from much farther away, but for now, the proximity will help you build the skill of sweeping.

4. Imagine beams of white light emanating from your fingers and penetrating an inch or two into your subject's body (Photo 7–b). The depth of your scanning is determined by intent. Keep your tongue on the roof of your mouth and continue with pranic breathing as you sweep.

5. Keeping your hands together, sweep slowly down the center of your subject's body, from the top of the head (crown), down through the face, the neck, chest, torso, and genitals and down the legs to the feet (Photo 7–c). You can determine for yourself how slowly each sweep should be as you become more proficient, but for now, 10 to 15 seconds per pass is a good rule of thumb. As you sweep, be aware of any heavy, sticky, or depressed feelings you might sense with your hands.

6. You may want to imagine the light beams scraping off dark, grayish-brown muddy material that sticks to the beams as they move downward.

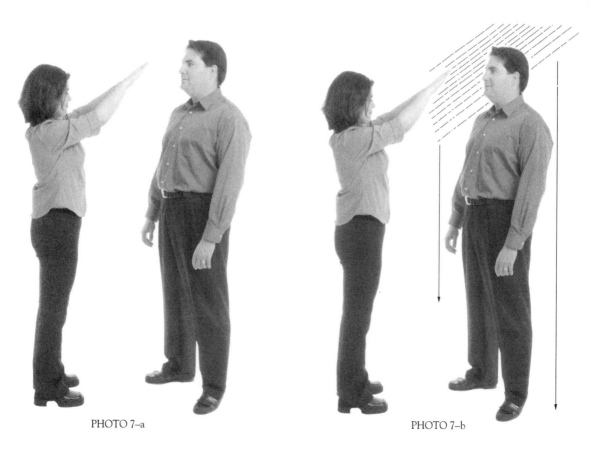

PHOTO 7–a   PHOTO 7–b

7. As you sweep past the feet, pull your hands away and flick the dirty energy in your hands briskly toward the salt water. You may want to visualize the dark material being thrown into the salt water. Some people even see it making a small splash. This constitutes the first of your five sweeps down the front of the body.

8. For the second pass, bring your hands back up to the starting position. Aim your hands above your subject's head, but separate them by about one and a half hand-widths. Sweep down the front of the body from head to toe with the same graceful motion (Photo 7–d). Be aware of any feelings of energetic disturbances. As you sweep past the feet, again flick the dirty energy into the salt water.

9. After every two sweeps, give your hands a spray or two from your alcohol bottle. It's okay if your hands drip as you sweep.

10. To begin your third pass, once again bring your hands back to the starting position. Aim them above your subject's head, and separate them three hand-widths. Then sweep down as you did on the first and second passes.

11. To begin your fourth pass, once again bring your hands back to the starting position. Aim your hands above your subject's head and separate them by roughly four and a half hand-widths. Sweep down, and then spray your hands with alcohol afterward.

12. For the fifth and final pass down the front of the body, have your subject spread his arms slightly (Photo 7–e). On this fifth sweep, your hands, or the beams you visualize emanating from them, will trace the outline of your subject's body. Put your hands in the beginning sweeping posture, pointing above the subject's head, then rotate them inward so that the backs of your hands and fingers are touching. It will be the same hand posture you would use if you were going to spread open a set of curtains with both hands.

13. From this position, sweep down the perimeter of the body. Sweep downward around the head, over the ears and shoulders, and down the outside of the slightly outstretched arms. Then sweep up the inside of the arms (the only time you will sweep upward) to the armpit. At the armpit begin sweeping downward again, tracing along the outside of the body and the legs down to the feet. Finish by flicking your hands into the salt water and then spraying them with alcohol.

14. Next, sweep the back of the aura. Ask your subject to bring her arms back to her sides and to turn around (or, you can walk around her until you're facing her back).

15. In the beginning, it may be helpful for you to reemphasize your intent occasionally by declaring that you now intend to "sweep so-and-so's back." If at any time, you feel like you need to recharge your sensitivity, take a few pranic breaths or repeat the Hand Sensitivity or the Presweeping Hand Preparation Exercise.

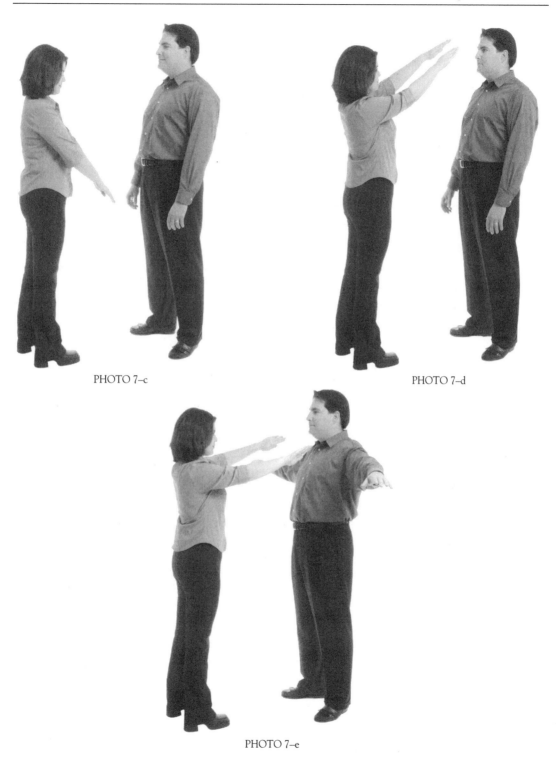

PHOTO 7–c

PHOTO 7–d

PHOTO 7–e

16. Sweep your subject's back with five head-to-toe passes as you did the front. Your fifth sweep on the back will also be with your subject's arms slightly spread.
17. Scan your subject's aura again. Note if it seems more balanced now.
18. When you are finished, cut the cord between you and your subject (Figure 7–6).
19. Conclude the exercise by shaking your hands and spraying them with alcohol again. Take a couple of pranic breaths and relax.

You may want to mention your impressions of any stickiness, heaviness, or depressions in the energy aura. If these coincide with an existing physical ailment your subject has told you about, use that as positive reinforcement. If you have no impressions, that's fine, too. You may also want to ask your subject how he feels. If he feels any more relaxed or calm, use that for positive reinforcement that you're sweeping properly; if not, that's fine. Even during the first general sweeping exercise, many subjects feel tangible results because you pass through several areas that are commonly tense and congested: the front and back heart and solar plexus chakras, and the chest and stomach.

You may find it beneficial to scan and sweep different people to compare their auras and any areas of energetic congestion.

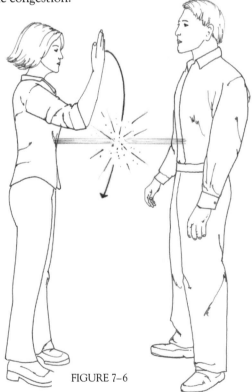

FIGURE 7–6

Sweeping to Heal a Burn

"Shortly after I had learned Pranic Healing, my mother splattered grease all over her arm while cooking. I began sweeping her entire arm, and within seconds, I noticed the redness diminishing. My mother reported that the pain was going away, too. When I stopped for 15 minutes, the redness started getting darker again. I started a cycle of sweeping for several minutes and resting for 20 minutes. After two hours it looked like she never had the burn. When I asked Grandmaster Choa later why the redness kept returning, he said it was because the heat's energy was deep inside the skin and that layers and layers of this heat energy were being literally 'excavated' as I swept."

—*Master Stephen Co*

GENERAL SWEEPING OF THE HEALTH RAYS OF ANOTHER PERSON

The health aura, a collection of foot-long energy rays that flow from our pores, needs healthful maintenance just as much as the inner aura and the chakras. The health aura acts as a "psychic shield," protecting you from other people's negative emotions and thoughts. When you are physically sick, your health rays are weak and drooping, and you are more susceptible to contamination by other people's negative energy, emotions, and thoughts. Having a strong health aura is essential for your physical, mental, and emotional well-being. You keep your health aura strong by sweeping or "combing" the health rays with the same two-handed general sweeping posture but with one minor variation: you sweep not with the fingers tight but with the fingers open and extended (Figure 7–7). Other than that, the sequence is almost exactly the same as general sweeping. Sweeping the health rays is a follow-up technique to general scanning rather than a stand-alone technique. Thus, after you perform general sweeping (Exercise 7–B) on your subject, continue with these steps. There is no need to perform the preparation steps if you sweep the health rays right after general sweeping.

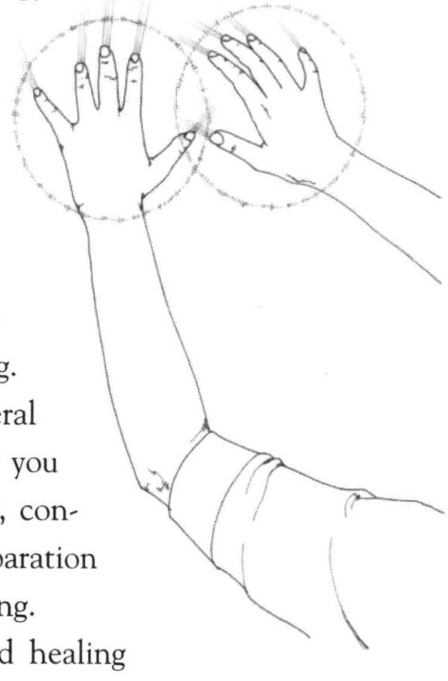

Straightening the health rays can have a very rapid healing effect. In class, students are instructed to stand and stretch their back

FIGURE 7–7

to determine how tight it feels before practicing general sweeping and straightening of the health rays. After only 5 minutes of general sweeping and straightening the health rays, nearly all students report that their backs feel more relaxed, and those who had any back pain report that it is substantially reduced.

Straightening the health rays can also have a very relaxing effect. Pranic Healing student Karla Alvarez was performing general sweeping and straightening the health rays for a woman who wanted simply to relieve her stress. After a few minutes, the woman fell fast asleep. She awoke 10 minutes later refreshed and relaxed.

EXERCISE 7–C: *General Sweeping of the Health Rays of Another Person*

If necessary, reestablish your intent by silently declaring to yourself that you intend to sweep and clean away the dirty prana from this person's health aura.

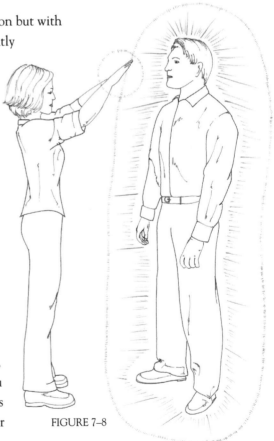

1. With hands in the general sweeping position but with the fingers spread, aim your fingers slightly above your subject's head. If you are standing about 3 feet away, your hands should be 4 to 6 inches from your subject's body.

2. Imagine beams of white light emanating from your spread fingers and penetrating an inch or two into your subject's body.

3. Now, slowly comb down the center of your subject's body, from the top of the head (crown), down through the face, the neck, chest, torso, and genitals, and down the legs to the feet (Figure 7–8). (*Note:* Comb but do not claw. Clawing is a more aggressive motion that can disrupt a person's energy. You make this distinction through intent and hand motion. Keep your intent on combing and use a smooth, gentle sweeping motion.) The pace you used in general scanning, 10 to 15 seconds per pass, is good. Remember to keep your

FIGURE 7–8

tongue on the roof of your mouth, and continue with pranic breathing as you sweep.

4. As you comb, be aware of any energetic disturbances: feelings of heaviness, stickiness, or depression.

5. If you wish, visualize that light beams are raking through the health rays and straightening them, as they comb out dark grayish-brown muddy material.

6. As you sweep past the feet, pull your hands away and flick the dirty energy briskly into the salt water. This constitutes the first of your five sweeps down the front of the body.

7. Continue as you did in general sweeping, moving your hands up above the head, separating them about one and a half hand-widths, and combing down again. After every two sweeps, spray your hands with alcohol. For the fifth and final pass down the front of the body, rake your subject with his arms spread slightly.

8. Now comb your subject's health rays from the back. Flick your hands into the salt water after each sweep, and spray them with alcohol after every two passes.

9. Scan your subject's aura again. Note if it seems more balanced now.

10. When you are finished, cut the cord between you and your subject.

11. Conclude the exercise by shaking your hands and spraying them with alcohol again. Take a few pranic breaths and relax.

If you swept the health rays of your subject immediately after performing general scanning on him, you may want to ask again how he feels and give him your impressions.

LOCAL SWEEPING OF ANOTHER PERSON

In local sweeping, you use the dog-paddle hand motion for small areas or joints, and the counterclockwise corkscrew hand motion for chakras. As with general scanning, it is helpful to practice on a subject with a known though simple health problem. A headache, stiff neck, sinus congestion, or sore knee are all good to work on.

EXERCISE 7–D: *Local Sweeping of Another Person—Specific Areas and Joints*

Stand for this exercise. Your warm-up is the same as that for Exercise 7–B. Then proceed.

1. Scan your targeted or agreed-upon area from several angles. If your subject has a sinus problem, for instance, scan in directly in front of the face, then maybe from each side of

the face near the cheekbones. If she has an inflamed knee, scan all four sides. Note your impressions of any energetic disturbances: bulges, heaviness, stickiness, or depressions.

2. Reestablish your intent by silently declaring to yourself that you intend to sweep and clean away the dirty prana from this area. Remember to keep your tongue on the roof of your mouth and continue with pranic breathing as you sweep.

3. With your dominant hand in the slightly cupped sweeping position and 4 to 6 inches from the area, begin sweeping with the dog-paddle motion, in short, brisk movements, down and away from the person's body, and down and away from you (Figure 7–9). One second per sweep is a good pace. Cover the entire target area with your sweeping, beginning at the left end of the area and moving to the right. Maintain a slight overlap as your sweeping strokes move from the left end to the right. If you're sweeping a large area, such as the stomach, you can make up to 10 sweeps with minimal overlap. If it's a smaller area, such as a knee or elbow, sweep the same area several times. For these small

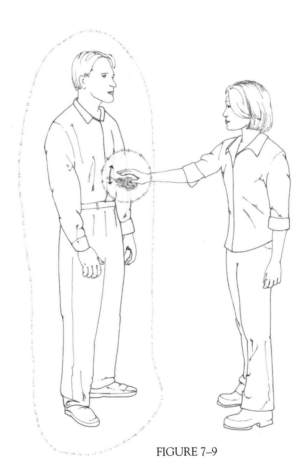

FIGURE 7–9

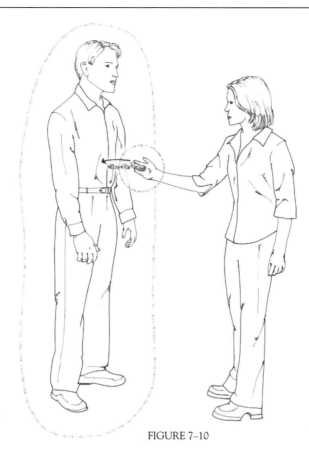

FIGURE 7–10

areas, double or triple up your sweeping passes; sweep down in the same groove two or three times before moving on.

4. As you sweep, be alert to feelings of heaviness, stickiness, or depression you might feel in your hands. Zero in on any you find and remove them by reinforcing your intent and sweeping through those areas with more will.

5. Add visualization, if you wish. See light beams extending from your fingers and penetrating several inches below the skin to scrape out grayish-brown dirty energy.

6. After 10 or so downward sweeps, you may wish to add an accumulation sweep, which is a horizontal sweep that cleans the dirty prana swept downward (Figure 7–10).

7. Regardless of the size of the target area, and whether or not you use the accumulation sweep, after 10 sweeps, pull your hand down and away and flick it toward the salt water.

8. Sweep the area again with 10 passes, moving left to right across the area, use the accumulation sweep if you wish, then flick the dirty prana into the salt water. Spray your hands with alcohol after every two sets of 10 passes.

9. Repeat this sequence of two sets of 10 passes four more times, which will give you a

total of 100 sweeps of the area.

10. If at any time you feel like you're losing your intent or hand sensitivity, take a break, walk around, and do the appropriate exercises.

11. Rescan the area to see if the energetic disturbance has been alleviated.

12. Cut the cord when you are finished.

13. Conclude the exercise by shaking your hands and spraying them with alcohol again. Take a few pranic breaths and relax.

Ask your subject how the area or problem feels. Is the pain reduced? Is the discomfort lessened? If the answer is yes, use it for positive reinforcement. If there appears to be no change, that's fine, too. If you'd like to address the problem further and your subject is willing, you may wish to try another 100 sweeps of the area.

Local Sweeping Stops Bleeding

"I got called into the emergency room one evening to treat a woman who came in passing large amounts of bright red blood and clots in her urine. She had presented several months earlier with advanced bladder cancer. This cancer had already metastasized to other parts of her body, so the bladder was left in, and now the tumor was bleeding profusely. What we normally do in a case like this is to place a large catheter into the bladder to remove the clots, then run saline solution into the bladder. This usually stops the bleeding. I performed this procedure, but the woman continued to bleed, so the next step was to operate to control the bleeding. I had the operating room crew called in. While we were waiting for her to be taken to the operating room, I scanned the woman and noted that there was thick, congested, dirty energy over her sex chakra. I thought, 'How can she possibly heal or stop bleeding with dirty congested energy in the bladder area?' I silently invoked and began sweeping the dirty energy away from her pelvis. I instructed the woman to do pranic breathing. Within 5 minutes, the bleeding completely stopped, and the urine remained clear for the next 24 hours. She was discharged the next day, and never had to have that particular operation."

—*Eric B. Robins, M.D.*

EXERCISE 7–E: *Local Sweeping of Another Person—Chakras*

For this exercise, you'll use the front solar plexus chakra as your target.

Stand for this exercise. Your warm-up is the same as that for Exercise 7–B. Then proceed.

1. Scan your subject's front solar plexus chakra and note any energetic disturbances.

2. Reestablish your intent by silently declaring to yourself that you intend to sweep and clean away the dirty prana from the front solar plexus. Remember to keep your tongue on the roof of your mouth and continue with pranic breathing as you sweep.

3. With your dominant hand in the slightly cupped sweeping position and 4 to 6 inches from your subject's front solar plexus chakra, begin sweeping with a tight counterclockwise motion of the wrist in sets of five (Figure 7–11). Remember how to determine counterclockwise: It is as if a clock facing outward were on the body part on which you are working. One second per revolution is a good pace. After five revolutions, pull your hand down and away and flick it into the salt water. After every two sets of five sweeps (10 total), spray your hand with alcohol.

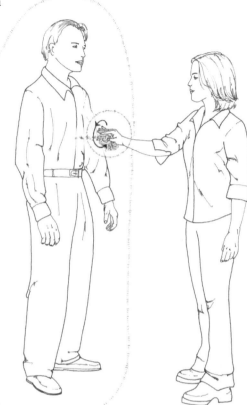

FIGURE 7–11

4. As you sweep, be aware of any heavy or sticky feelings. Even though a chakra is a smaller target than an arm, a leg, or the torso, there can still be pockets of congestion within the chakra. Zero in on any you find, and remove them by reinforcing your intent and sweeping through those areas with more will.

5. Add visualization, if you wish. See light beams extending from your fingers and penetrating several inches into the chakra to scrape out grayish-brown dirty energy.

6. Repeat this sequence of two sets of five counterclockwise twists five more times, which will give you a total of 60 sweeps of the front solar plexus chakra.

7. If at any time you feel like you're losing your intent or hand sensitivity, take a break, walk around, and do the appropriate exercises.

8. Rescan the front solar plexus chakra to see if there's been any reduction in the amount of congestion.

9. Cut the cord when you are finished.

10. Conclude the exercise by shaking your hands and spraying them with alcohol again. Take a few pranic breaths and relax.

Since the front solar plexus chakra is the seat of the expressed emotions and is frequently congested when we're stressed, sweeping it often quickly produces a state of relaxation. If the person says he's less tense afterwards, use that for positive reinforcement. If there appears to be no change, that's fine, too.

You may wish to scan and sweep other chakras or a few other people for comparison.

Local Sweeping of Chakras Relieves Emotionally Caused Physical Pain

"While teaching a class in Houston, I asked for a volunteer with back pain. A woman came forward and demonstrated to the whole class that she could bend forward only about 20 degrees. After 5 minutes of general sweeping, she was able to touch the floor with her hands. On the last day of the class I was performing a follow-up treatment on her, with local sweeping of each individual chakra. When I swept her back solar plexus chakra, she started screaming at the top of her lungs "NO!" and began running around the room. She came back, and I continued sweeping her whole aura, but especially the front and back solar plexus chakras. She calmed down, and her facial expression changed, as if a whole lifetime of troubles had been lifted off her shoulders. We asked her what happened, and she replied that she had been harboring a horrible emotional trauma: When she was a child, her mom tried to kill her so she wouldn't have to suffer with the rest of the family in a concentration camp. This had left an emotional scar that lasted for over fifty years and manifested physically as back pain. Sweeping removed the dirty emotional energy—and the trauma— that she had not been able to remove with any other treatment she tried. The next day her friends and family were amazed at the transformation. They said she looked like a completely different person!"

—*Master Stephen Co*

GENERAL SELF-SWEEPING

You can choose between two different ways to perform general self-sweeping. The first, Exercise 7–F, is a full visualization technique in which you perform the 10-sweep routine that you used in Exercise 7–B, on yourself. The second, Exercise 7–G, involves less visualization and a slightly different routine that has you using the dog-paddle motion on your energy body. They're both equally effective. See which works better for you.

EXERCISE 7–F: *General Self-Sweeping—10-Sweep Routine*

You may sit or stand for this exercise. Your warm-up is the same as that for Exercise 7–B, except you don't have a subject to query about any existing health problems. Then proceed.

1. Establish a quick energetic baseline for yourself. Note the relative shape and strength of your aura, as well as any areas of congestion or depletion.
2. If necessary, reestablish your intent by silently declaring to yourself that you intend to sweep and clean away the dirty prana from your energy body.
3. Visualize yourself about 2 to 3 feet in front of you, using your preferred technique. Remember you can increase identification with the visualization by saying your name three times. Remember to keep your tongue on the roof of your mouth and continue with pranic breathing as you sweep.
4. With your hands in the slightly cupped general sweeping position and with the forefingers and inside edge of your hands touching, aim your fingers slightly above the head of your visualized body.
5. Imagine beams of white light emanating from your fingers and penetrating an inch or two into your visualized body.
6. Follow the sequence used in general sweeping of another person on this visualization of yourself.
7. After every two sweeps, spray your hands with alcohol.
8. After you complete sweeping the front of your visualized figure, turn it around and sweep the back.
9. After you complete the back, rescan your aura. Note if it seems more balanced now. Note, also, if you feel lighter, more relaxed, or more refreshed.
10. Conclude the exercise by shaking your hands and spraying them with alcohol again. Take a few pranic breaths and relax.

EXERCISE 7–G: *General Self-Sweeping—Dog-Paddle Routine*

For this routine, it is better if you stand. Begin with the warm-up and steps 1 and 2 from Exercise 7–F, then proceed.

1. With your hands in the slightly cupped general sweeping position, place your hands just above your head at the crown.
2. Imagine your hands surrounded by a paddle of bright white light. You'll sweep with the

inside (the thumb side) of your hands. Remember to keep your tongue on the roof of your mouth and continue with pranic breathing as you sweep.

3. Dog-paddle down the center line of your body, from your crown down to your feet (Figure 7–12). It's okay if you bend at the waist or at the knees as you sweep through your legs. As you pass through your feet, throw the dirty energy into the salt water.

4. For your second pass, bring your hands back above your head but slightly to the left, so that they follow a head-to-toe path roughly from the left side of your head down through the left side of your torso and your left leg, down to your feet. Throw the dirty energy into the salt water and spray your hands with alcohol.

5. For the third sweep, begin with your hands roughly over your left shoulder and sweep downward with the dog paddle motion. After you pass the feet, throw the dirty energy into the salt water and spray your hands with alcohol.

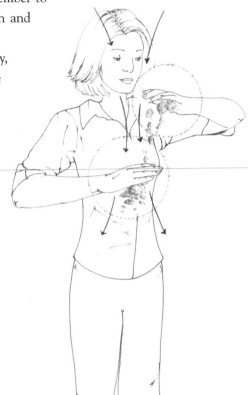

FIGURE 7–12

6. Repeat this sequence for the right side of your body.

7. Then, using your preferred visualization method, dog-paddle-sweep the back of your energy body in the same way: once down the center line and then twice to the left and twice to the right.

8. After you complete the back, rescan your aura. Note if it seems more balanced now. See also if you feel lighter, more relaxed, or more refreshed.

9. Conclude the exercise by shaking your hands and spraying them with alcohol again. Take a few pranic breaths and relax.

A few minutes of general sweeping after you return home in the evening is a great way to pick yourself up at the end of a long, stressful day. Pranic Healing student Naila Vavra uses this technique frequently. She describes one particular day when she felt "exhausted and drained," her back was "tense," and she was "emotionally upset." But after ten minutes of general sweeping, she says, "My back was relaxed, my emotions were clear, and I was ready to go out for dinner. I was actually astounded at how quickly my body reacted to general sweeping."

GENERAL SELF-SWEEPING OF YOUR HEALTH RAYS

This technique is a combination of general sweeping of another person's health rays with your preferred visualization technique. Remember, sweeping your health rays is a follow-up or supplement to general scanning rather than a stand-alone technique.

EXERCISE 7–H: *General Self-Sweeping of Your Health Rays*

Stand for this exercise. Your warm-up is the same as that for Exercise 7–B, except you don't have a subject to query about existing health problems. We'll refer to this sequence from now on as your "standard warm-up." Then proceed.

1. Using your preferred visualization method and with your hands slightly cupped and fingers spread, aim your fingers slightly above your visualization of yourself.
2. Imagine beams of white light emanating from your spread fingers and penetrating an inch or two into your visualization. Remember to keep your tongue on the roof of your mouth, and continue with pranic breathing as you sweep.
3. Slowly comb down the center of your visualized body, from the top of the head (crown), through the face, the neck, chest, torso, and genitals, and down the legs to the feet. Remember to comb but do not claw. If you wish, add the visualization that the light beams are raking through the health rays and straightening them, as they comb out dark grayish-brown muddy material.
4. As you comb, be aware of any heavy or sticky feelings your hands detect. Reinforce your intent, and comb through them with a little more force. As you sweep past the feet, pull your hands away and flick them briskly into the salt water.
5. Continue combing your visualization with five strokes down the front and five down the back. For the fifth and final pass down both sides of the body, rake your visualization with arms spread slightly.

6. Rescan your aura, or take a quick energetic baseline measurement. Note if it's more balanced now.

7. Conclude the exercise by shaking your hands and spraying them with alcohol again. Take a few pranic breaths, and relax.

LOCAL SELF-SWEEPING

This technique combines local sweeping on another person with your preferred visualization technique. There are two ways to do local self-sweeping: full visualization or partial visualization. Since you already encountered these options in scanning, we include them as self-sweeping variants rather than two different exercises. With *full visualization*, you perform all your self-sweeping on a visualization of yourself, even when working on an area that you can reach with your sweeping hand. With *partial visualization*, you use visualization only on those areas that you cannot reach with your sweeping hand.

For example, if you are right-hand-dominant and you have a pain in your left shoulder, with full visualization you'd imagine a vivid picture of yourself across from you and then work on that image. With partial visualization you'd reach across your body and actually do the sweeping on the left shoulder with your right hand. Of course, for the back and the back chakras you would always have to use visualization. As with all variations and options, experiment and see which is more effective. Finally, if you do have an existing condition, such as a sore knee or elbow, or stomach discomfort, feel free to use it as a target in this exercise.

EXERCISE 7–1: *Local Self-Sweeping—Specific Areas and Joints*

Sit or stand for this exercise. Perform your standard warm-up.

1. Scan your target area from a couple of angles to get a sense of any energetic disturbances.

2. If necessary, reestablish your intent by silently declaring to yourself that you intend to sweep and clean away the dirty prana from this particular area. Remember to keep your tongue on the roof of your mouth, and continue with pranic breathing as you sweep.

3. With your dominant hand in the slightly cupped sweeping position and 4 to 6 inches from the area, begin sweeping with a dog-paddle motion, in short brisk movements,

down and away from the area. You can use the entire edge of your hand, not just the fingers.

4. One second per sweep is a good pace. Cover the entire target area with your sweeping, beginning at the left end of the area and moving to the right. Maintain a slight overlap as your sweeping strokes move from left to right. If it's a small area, such as a knee or elbow, go over the same area several times; double up or triple up your passes.

5. As you sweep, be aware of any heavy or sticky feelings. Zero in on any you find, and remove them by reinforcing your intent and sweeping through those areas with more will.

6. After 10 or so downward sweeps, add the accumulation sweep, if you wish.

7. Regardless of the size of the target and whether or not you use the accumulation sweep, after 10 sweeps, pull your hand down and away and flick it into the salt water. Now go back and sweep the area again with 10 passes, moving left to right across the area, add the accumulation sweep, if you wish, then flick the dirty prana into the salt water. Spray your hands with alcohol after every two sets of 10 passes.

8. Repeat this sequence of two sets of 10 passes four more times, for a total of 100 sweeps.

9. Rescan the area to see if any energetic congestion has been diminished.

10. Conclude the exercise by shaking your hands and spraying them with alcohol again. Take a few pranic breaths and relax.

Assess the area or problem. How does it feel? If you had any pain or discomfort, has it been reduced? If the answer is yes, use it for positive reinforcement. If there appears to be no change, that's fine, too. If you wish to work on the area again, repeat the exercise, sweeping it another 100 times.

Local Sweeping to "Heal the Healers"

"Many massage therapists come to my Pranic Healing workshops. When I ask how many of them experience recurring arm and shoulder pain, nearly all raise their hands. I then ask for the one with the worst pain and proceed to sweep the person's arm and shoulder. After about 5 minutes of local sweeping of the arms, shoulders, and armpits, the pain is usually completely gone. This pain usually results from repetitive motion and accumulation of dirty energy absorbed during their sessions with clients."

—*Master Stephen Co*

EXERCISE 7–J: *Local Self-Sweeping—Chakras*

For the sake of consistency with the previous exercises, and because it's easy to reach, we'll learn how to self-sweep your front solar plexus chakra.

Sit or stand for this exercise. Perform your standard warm-up, and then decide if you're going to use visualization.

1. Scan your front solar plexus chakra, and note any energetic disturbances.
2. Reestablish your intent by silently declaring to yourself that you intend to sweep and clean away the dirty prana from the front solar plexus. Remember to keep your tongue on the roof of your mouth, and continue with pranic breathing as you sweep.
3. If you're going to self-sweep without visualization, turn your dominant hand backward so that your fingers are pointing at your front solar plexus chakra from 4 to 6 inches away. If you're using full visualization, imagine your fingertips 4 to 6 inches from your visualized body. Whether you use visualization or not, your fingers should be in the slightly cupped sweeping position. You sweep either your actual body or your visualization in a counterclockwise motion. Remember how to determine your counterclockwise orientation: Imagine a clock with its face outward lying on the body part on which you are working. This applies to working both on your physical body and on a visualization of your body.
4. Begin sweeping with a tight counterclockwise motion of the wrist. One second per revolution is a good pace. Visualize light beams if you wish.
5. After five revolutions, pull your hand down and away and flick it into the salt water. After every two sets of five sweeps, spray your hand with alcohol.
6. As you sweep, be aware of any heavy or sticky feelings your hand detects. Even though a chakra is a much smaller target than an arm, a leg, or an entire vertical section of the body, there can still be pockets within the perimeter of a chakra. Zero in on any you find, and remove them by reinforcing your intent and sweeping through those areas with a bit more will.
7. Repeat this sequence of two sets of five counterclockwise twists five more times, which will give you a total of 60 sweeps of the front solar plexus chakra.
8. Rescan your front solar plexus chakra to see if there's been any reduction in the amount of congestion.
9. Conclude the exercise by shaking your hands and spraying them with alcohol again. Take a couple of pranic breaths, and relax.

The front solar plexus chakra is the seat of many of our negative emotions. A thorough sweeping of the area should bring about a calm, relaxed feeling. If you do feel more relaxed, use it for positive reinforcement. If there appears to be no change, that's fine, too. If you wish to work on your front solar plexus chakra again, repeat the exercise. You may also wish to scan and sweep other chakras.

A Few Final Notes on Sweeping

- You can't sweep too much or overclean. If anything, people sweep too little. *Effective energy healing is 75 to 80 percent cleaning.* As you will learn in the next chapter, however, you must be careful when energizing because you can overcharge an area or chakra, which may create congestion or aggravate an existing condition. In the step-by-step energetic remedies you will learn, the ratio of sweeping to energizing is four or five or even more to one. Thus, you sweep the area or chakra 40 or 50 times or even more, then energize it for 10 cycles of pranic breathing.

- Here are some sweeping visualization tips: When you visualize the light around your scanning hand, imagine your hand as a Ping-Pong paddle or spatula, or as if it were inserted into an oven mitt. See a flat oval-shaped field of light all around your hand. You could also visualize your hand as a garden trowel, which has a more elongated shape. You may supplement these or any other visualization by thinking of the light field as being like flypaper, with dirty energy sticking to it as you sweep away.

- You can supercharge your sweeping ability by placing one drop of lavender oil and five drops of baby oil on your palm and rubbing it in before you scan and sweep. Or, mix up a small bottle of those two oils in that same 1:5 ratio for more frequent use. As you will find out in Chapter 10, lavender oil has strong cleansing properties. If you use lavender oil, continue to spray with alcohol as you normally would. If the oil begins to wash off, simply reapply it.

SWEEPING CHECKLIST

Here is a summary of the key steps in sweeping, indexed according to the technique:

Standard Warm-Up:

1. Roll up your sleeves, take off your shoes and belt, and empty your pockets.
2. Place your tongue on the roof of your mouth.

3. Do pranic breathing.
4. Tap your heart chakra.
5. Do Hand Sensitivity Exercise 1 or 2.
6. Have your bowl of salt water and alcohol sprayer handy.
7. Perform Presweeping Hand Preparation Exercise 7–A, including invocation.
8. If working/practicing on someone else:
    - Ask subject if she has any current health problems.
    - Tell subject to keep her tongue on the roof of her mouth.
    - Cut cords after the session.
    - Get feedback after session.

General Self-Sweeping (10-Sweep with Both Hands Cupped):

1. Scan the aura at several points to determine the general energy level.
2. First do a head-to-toe sweep down the center line, using visualization if you wish.
3. Flick the dirty prana into salt water.
4. For second head-to-toe-sweep, separate your hands by a one to one and a half hand-widths.
5. Flick the dirty prana into salt water.
6. Spray your hands with alcohol.
7. Continue sweeping, maintaining slight overlap as you move hands outward by one to one and a half hand-widths each time.
8. Spray hands with alcohol after every two passes.
9. On fifth and final sweep, with arms slightly outstretched, trace outline of body.
10. Repeat on back.

General Self-Sweeping (Dog Paddle):

1. Scan the aura at several points to determine the general energy level.
2. Do the first head-to-toe sweep down the center line, using dog-paddle motion.
3. Flick dirty prana into salt water.
4. Move hands to left side of head and sweep down front of body.
5. Flick the dirty prana into salt water.
6. Spray your hands with alcohol.
7. Move your hands to just over the left shoulder and sweep down the front of the body.

8. Repeat dog-paddle sweeps down the right side of the body.
9. Spray your hands with alcohol after every two passes.
10. Repeat on back, using visualization.

General Self-Sweeping of Health Rays (With Both Hands, Fingers Spread and Extended):

1. Perform general sweeping first.
2. Rescan the aura to determine the level of energetic congestion.
3. Do the first head-to-toe sweep down the center line with a combing motion, using visualization if you wish.
4. Flick the dirty prana into salt water.
5. For the second head-to-toe-sweep, separate your hands by one to one and a half hand-widths.
6. Flick the dirty prana into salt water.
7. Spray your hands with alcohol.
8. Continue combing, maintaining a slight overlap as you move your hands outward by one to one and a half hand-widths each time.
9. Spray your hands with alcohol after every two passes.
10. On fifth and final sweep, with the hands slightly outstretched, trace the outline of the body.
11. Repeat on back.

Local Self-Sweeping of Joint or Small Body Area (With One Hand, Usually the Dominant Hand):

1. Scan the target to determine the level of energetic congestion.
2. Do a first set of five to ten dog paddles, using visualization if you wish.
3. Flick the dirty prana into salt water.
4. Do a second set of five to ten dog paddles.
5. Flick the dirty prana into salt water.
6. Spray your hand with alcohol.
7. Continue sweeping and then scanning periodically until scanning reveals that area is clean.
8. Spray your hand with alcohol after every two passes.

Local Self-Sweeping of a Chakra (with One Hand, Usually the Dominant Hand):

1. Scan the target chakra to determine the level of energetic congestion.
2. Do a first set of five counterclockwise sweeps. (Remember how to determine your counterclockwise orientation: Whether you use visualization or turn your hand backwards to sweep your actual body, it is as if a watch with its face outward is lying on the part of the body on which you are working.)
3. Flick the dirty prana into salt water.
4. Do a second set of five counterclockwise sweeps.
5. Flick the dirty prana into salt water.
6. Spray your hand with alcohol.
7. Continue sweeping and then scanning periodically until scanning reveals that the area is clean.
8. Spray your hand with alcohol after every two passes.

SIX STEPS DAILY PRACTICE ROUTINE—UPDATE

As needed:

1. *Direct clearing* (Exercises 3–A and 3–B).
2. *Stretching and loosening the diaphragm* (Exercises 4–A).
3. *Hand Sensitivity Exercises 1 and 2* (Exercises 1–A and 5–A).

Daily practice:

4. *Pranic breathing* (Exercise 4–B). Use your preferred rhythm and retention sequence.
5. *General scanning* (Exercises 5–B to 5–E). Practice on a variety of targets: your arm, your leg, and other parts of your body; plants, animals, and other people; energetic baseline.
6. *Specific scanning.* Practice on small targets (for example, your left wrist or right ear); individual chakras (Exercises 6–A and 6–B); chakral baseline (Exercise 6–E); self-scanning using visualization (Exercise 6–C); specific scanning with your nondominant hand (the hand with which you don't normally scan); specific scanning with both hands simultaneously.
7. *Sweeping* (Exercises 7–B to 7–J). General sweeping of another person, general self-sweeping, sweeping health rays of another person, self-sweeping health rays, sweeping chakras of another person, self-sweeping chakras.

By this time, you should have a better sense of your aptitude for these exercises, the personal areas on which you need to focus, and the time you wish to devote to this work. Your practice should become more individualized. Cut down your time on the basic techniques and spend more time scanning and sweeping.

In the next chapter, you'll learn the third energy manipulation technique, *energizing*.

CHAPTER 8

Pump It Up—
Energizing Areas
of Depletion

"I have tried a few different types of healing techniques in the past few years, but none has been so clearly powerful as Pranic Healing. The energy that moves through you while performing a healing is incredible. I find it easy to work with because it is not left up to intuition. There is a step-by-step guide to follow for different healing needs. Practicing this healing on others and myself has helped to move my life in so many wonderful ways. I am forever grateful for the privilege of being introduced to this extremely powerful healing method."

—ELIZABETH SMITH, LAKEVILLE, MINNESOTA

After scanning for energetic disturbances in your aura and sweeping them away, you must replenish the now-clean area with fresh prana. As you read in Chapter 1, we all have the baseline ability to assimilate life force and use it; your body knows instinctively how to produce and use prana for healing. But you can accelerate the body's healing process through *energizing*, the Pranic Healing method of generating great quantities of high-quality prana and then consciously directing it throughout your body. Energizing is the third of the three energy manipulation techniques.

The energizing procedure you learn here is a particularly effective method called the *water pump technique*. It utilizes *external generation*, which means you draw from the nearly limitless sources of prana from outside your body. External generation is easier to learn and more effective than *internal generation*, in which you build up your own personal supply of energy—usually through lengthy practice of complex meditations, extensive breathing, and physical exercises—and use that for healing. *Chi kung* and Taoist yoga are primarily internal-generation systems. While internal generation produces results, it runs down your personal energy battery, so you constantly have to recharge as you heal. You'll find it easier and quicker to learn to assimilate air, solar, and ground prana and utilize them for healing.

THE BASICS OF ENERGIZING WITH THE WATER PUMP TECHNIQUE

The Pranic Healing energizing system combines three external prana-generation techniques—*pranic breathing*, the *chakral technique*, and *divine invocation*—into one optimal method, the *water pump technique*.

The water pump is an optimal technique for four reasons:

- It's simple to learn. You can learn it in an hour and make it work within two weeks.
- It relies primarily on intent and reasonably good form and technique. You don't need perfect visualization skills to use it effectively.
- It draws on the nearly inexhaustible supply of prana in the air, the sun, and the ground. You do not need to deplete your own finite supply of prana.
- It utilizes all three methods of externally drawing in prana. You get the maximum amount of energy.

You begin the water pump technique by asking for divine guidance and the ability to draw in and utilize this gift of healing energy appropriately. This is the *divine invocation*. You then form your intent to draw in prana through a source chakra and to radiate it from the chakra of your projecting hand to your target. This is the *chakral technique*. Finally, you use rhythm and retention as you breathe to increase your capacity for energy. This is *pranic breathing*. Then you use your intent and visualization to project the prana to the depth you want and in the appropriate color. You'll learn about colored prana in the next chapter.

Proper Hand Position for Energizing

The correct hand posture for energizing is similar to the one you used for sweeping and scanning: arms relaxed, armpits open, and wrists loose. The receiving hand is palm up, extended slightly forward and away from the body. The projecting hand is held with the palm pointing slightly forward so that the hand chakra is aiming at your target (Figure 8–1). Prana can be projected over a significant distance. In fact, this technique can be used for

distant healing, in which you work on a visualization of someone who is not in the room with you. But initially, keep
your projecting hand 4 to 6 inches from the target.

In sweeping, you rotate the hand counterclockwise
to unscrew dirty energy. When you energize, you move
your projecting hand in a clockwise motion; this drives
the energy in. The principal is the same as acupuncture.
An acupuncturist twists needles clockwise to "strengthen
and tonify," and twists the needles counterclockwise to
"remove or unblock" an energy channel. You will use the
same method of determining clockwise orientation that
you used to determine counterclockwise orientation: place
or imagine a clock with its face outward lying on the body
part on which you are working, then follow the hands clockwise. This applies both to working on your physical body and to
working on a visualization of your body.

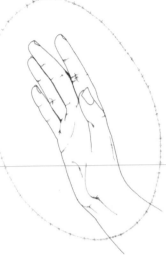

FIGURE 8–1

Sweeping Before Energizing

You *always* sweep before energizing, whether the area is congested or depleted. Sweeping
cleans out any residual dirty energy and helps prepare the area to absorb fresh prana.

It's like cleaning out a wound before changing the dressing and applying fresh medicine. You cannot overcleanse.

How Long to Energize?

As you become more experienced, you can rely on your ability to scan and feel for the
appropriate level of prana. When you feel a slight repulsion from the energized area or
chakra, or you feel that the prana in the deficient area is built up to a level where it seems
even with the contour of the nearby energetic anatomy, you're finished energizing. You may
develop an intuition that tells you, "That's enough prana." When you work on other people, you can rely on their feedback. If, for instance, you energize a person's front solar plexus
and your subject reports fullness or tightness in the chest, you've energized too much. The
remedy is simple: Sweep away the excess prana until it reaches the appropriate level in relation to the nearby energetic anatomy. Until you build up that level of experience and sensitivity, however, rely on this rule of thumb: Energize for five to seven cycles of pranic

breathing for simple ailments, such as a mild headaches, and 10 or more cycles for more difficult problems, such as a serious sprain. Scan periodically as you energize to determine if the area fills up before you reach the recommended number of breaths.

Feeling a Depleted Area Fill Up with Energy

"One of my bladder cancer patients was on the exam table awaiting a cystoscopy, which is a quick outpatient procedure where we look up into the patient's bladder with a lighted scope. As I walked into the room, I saw him squirming around on the table. I asked him if he was uncomfortable, and he replied that he had terrible lower back pain and spasms. Three years earlier he had undergone a double laminectomy to treat herniated disks, but his pain remained. Physical therapy hadn't helped, either. After the cystoscopy, I brought him to an exam room where I scanned his lower back and basic chakra and found them to be quite depleted of energy. After sweeping the area, I energized the lower back and the basic until I felt resistance, as if there were a spring pushing back against my palm. I also asked—as I always do—for the patient's feedback. The gentleman told me the pain was diminishing. That's how I know when I've energized an area or chakra sufficiently.

"By the way, I see this man frequently for his cancer, and the back pain has not returned in over 18 months."

—*Eric B. Robins, M.D.*

Stabilizing Projected Prana

Prana is fluid, and freshly projected prana is particularly fluid, so you need to stabilize it to make sure it stays where it is directed. After you complete an energizing technique and are satisfied that the formerly deficient area is now full, stabilize in one of two ways: Either form an intent that the prana stay there and say "stabilize" three times; or visualize yourself painting the area or chakra with light blue. (As you'll see in the next chapter, blue prana has a minimizing, slowing, or inhibiting effect.) You may simply imagine dipping your projecting hand into a can of light blue paint and then gently making three passes over the area.

PROGRESSIVE ENERGIZING EXERCISES

Even if you're only practicing the act of energizing, you must energize only areas that you have determined, through scanning, to be depleted of prana. If you project prana into an area or chakra that is already clean and full, you can create congestion. And if you project energy into an area or chakra that is already congested, you may aggravate the condition further. The energizing techniques we present here are powerful, so even a novice healer will project prana. We've had cases where beginners practicing on each other produced some startling, though unintended, results. One student was practicing projecting orange prana, which is a strong color used to break up and expel dirty energy, and he did so too willfully into the abdomen of another student. She developed diarrhea on the spot.

The people on whom you get permission to practice *must* have identifiable energetic deficiencies. If you don't have a human subject, and you have no energetic deficiencies yourself, you can still practice and learn energizing by projecting prana into a visualized generic human figure, or by projecting prana against a wall or a paper target on the wall.

Here is the sequence of progressive energizing exercises:

1. Simple projection: visualization practice.
2. Energizing depleted areas or chakras of another person using simple projection.
3. Energizing depleted areas or chakras of another person using the water pump technique.
4. Self-energizing your own depleted areas or chakras using the water pump technique.

As with scanning and sweeping, this is an *optimal* sequence for learning to energize properly. Do your best to follow the order of this sequence, but regular practice is more important than following these steps perfectly. The exercises include provisions for practicing without a partner (for example, projecting onto a wall or into an imaginary human figure).

If you have the fundamentals of scanning and sweeping down, you should be projecting prana consistently after two weeks of daily practice.

SIMPLE PROJECTION: VISUALIZATION PRACTICE

Though visualization is not critical to mastering the water pump technique, it does enhance your energizing effectiveness. Thus, we include this simple projection visualization exercise. You'll need a flashlight that projects a strong core of light at the center of its beam. Pelican flashlights, which have a halogen bulb and are used by scuba divers and fire departments, have a good, solid beam. Mag-Lites, the two- and three-cell flashlights used by police departments, are also good.

EXERCISE 8–A: *Visualization Practice*

1. In a room with the lights turned low, project the flashlight beam onto a white wall, or a white sheet of unlined paper that you've placed upon the wall. Hold the flashlight 2 to 3 feet from your target. This should produce a tight beam about 3 inches in diameter.
2. Observe the beam as it cuts through the dark and projects onto the wall (Figure 8–2). Study the beam and its solid core for 30 seconds.

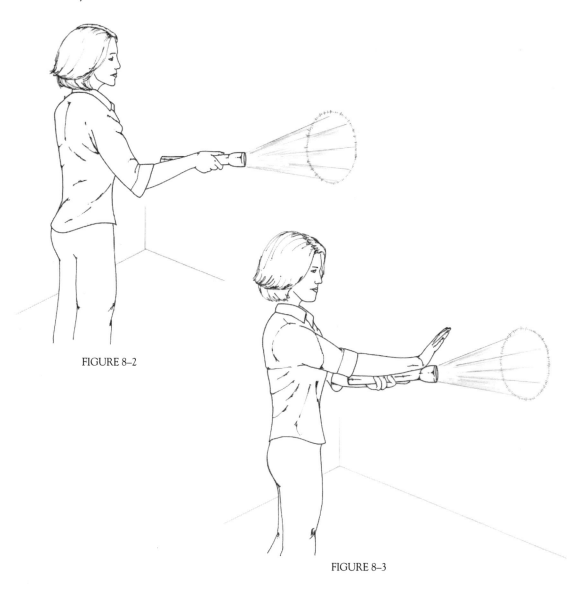

FIGURE 8–2

FIGURE 8–3

3. Put your projecting hand in the proper energy-projecting position. Hold the flashlight in your nondominant hand, and move it directly under your projecting hand (Figure 8–3).

4. Focus on the core of the beam on the wall and then trace it with your eyes back to the palm chakra of your projecting hand. Hold your attention on your palm chakra for a few moments, then trace the beam back to the wall, from your palm chakra to the white core of the beam on the wall. Trace this back and forth three times slowly.

5. Close your eyes. Keeping the flashlight in place, imagine that brilliant white light with the solid core flowing from your palm chakra. Hold this visualization for 10 seconds. Now open your eyes and trace the beam back and forth one more time. Then, close your eyes again and hold the visualization for 10 more seconds.

6. Relax, then repeat the exercise again.

Take your time with this exercise, which is designed purely to help you visualize. Have fun with it. After you practice a few times, try imagining that the head of the flashlight is actually *on* the center of your palm and projecting its beam directly from your palm chakra.

ENERGIZING DEPLETED AREAS OR CHAKRAS OF ANOTHER PERSON USING SIMPLE PROJECTION

This exercise enhances your ability to visualize projected prana. You imagine the energy on your target without regard to where it is coming from. Though not as strong an energizing technique as the water pump, simple projection still produces energy. Thus, to be safe, it's best that you practice only on verifiably depleted areas in your subject's energetic anatomy. You determine them through scanning. If you don't have a partner with whom to practice, work on a visualization of a generic human figure, or practice against a white wall.

EXERCISE 8–B: *Energizing Depleted Areas or Chakras of Another Person Using Simple Projection*

Both you and your subject should stand. Your subject should be about 3 feet away. Perform your standard warm-up (have your alcohol bottle and salt water container handy as part of your standard warm-up).

1. Begin with a general energetic baseline scan (Exercise 6–D): Scan the outside of both knees, the outside of both hips, both forearms, and the temples in sequence until you get a sense of your subject's energetic baseline. Then check any areas your subject indicates may be a problem—for example, a sprained ankle, a headache, a stiff neck, an upset stomach. Scan also the chakras associated with any identified problems (Table 1–I). If your subject reports no health problems, scan the front and back solar plexus chakras, the throat and the *ajna* (the chakras frequently congested or depleted with stress-related complaints), and the navel and the basic (the chakras frequently congested or depleted if general vitality is low). Even if your subject reports feeling fine, it would not be uncommon to find any of these chakras a little out of balance.

2. In any areas of energetic disturbance, whether they're congested or depleted, sweep the dirty prana away and dispose of it properly using salt water. Spray your hands with alcohol as necessary. Begin now in all your practice sessions to check the energetic condition of your target by scanning it periodically. After every 50 or so sweeps, take a break and scan the area to determine how much congestion you've swept away and how much remains.

3. Next, energize in this way: Put your projecting hand in the proper position 4 to 6 inches from your target area. Put your other hand at your side or in your pocket. Visualize a brilliant white beam of light radiating from your palm into the target area (Figure 8–4).

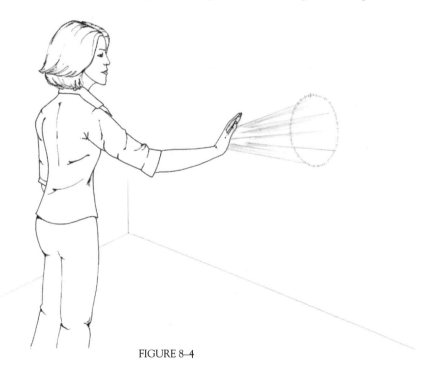

FIGURE 8–4

Continue with pranic breathing. To establish the visualization and to provide a visual frame of reference, remember how the beam of the flashlight looked as it was projected onto the wall. Trace the beam of prana from your palm chakra to the target and back a few times. See a brilliant white circle superimposed on the target.

4. If it's a small local area, such as a knee or a chakra, expand the white ring to encompass the width of the target. If it's a larger area, such as the stomach or the abdomen, move your energizing hand in left to right passes across the area so that you cover the entire area.

5. Rotate your hand in small clockwise circles occasionally as you project prana to drive the energy in. (Remember how to determine clockwise orientation.)

6. If you're working on a simple problem, continue for five to seven cycles of pranic breathing; 10 if the problem is more complex. Or energize until you feel that the area is full.

7. Break contact for a moment. Relax, shake your hands, and walk around for a few seconds.

8. Rescan the area to check the energy level. If the area still feels deficient, energize it further. Ask your subject how he feels, and make adjustments if necessary. For instance, if at any time the subject feels tightness or congestion, you've overenergized the area. Simply sweep away the excess energy until the subject feels better.

9. Continue work on any other areas of energetic disturbance: scan, sweep, then energize.

10. Cut the cord when you are finished.

11. Conclude by shaking your hands and spraying them with alcohol. Take a few pranic breaths and relax.

ENERGIZING THE DEPLETED AREAS OR CHAKRAS OF ANOTHER PERSON USING THE WATER PUMP TECHNIQUE

The instructions and admonitions from the previous exercise apply even more so here, since this is a more powerful technique. Perform it only on verifiably depleted areas in your subject's energetic anatomy. The water pump is the energizing technique for both large and small local areas, as well as chakras. During the water pump technique, it is very common to feel positive changes in your source chakra. People describe it as "warming up" or "opening up," as if siphoning in the energy.

EXERCISE 8–C: *Energizing the Depleted Areas or Chakras of Another Person Using the Water Pump Technique*

Perform your standard warm-up. Perform steps 1 and 2 from Exercise 8–B, then proceed.

1. Energize this way: Put your hands in the proper position, with your energy-projecting hand 4 to 6 inches from your target area and your receiving hand palm up and slightly in front and to the side of your body.

2. Place your awareness lightly on both palm chakras and form your intent to draw in air and solar prana through your receiving hand and to project this prana into the target area. Example: "I now intend to draw in prana through my left hand and project it from my right hand into ____." Begin pranic breathing, and as you do, keep light awareness on the receiving and projecting palm chakras. (*Note:* Don't correlate your pranic breathing with the intake and outflow of prana. Don't imagine that you're drawing in prana on your inbreath and beaming it outward on your outbreath. Our experiments show that this produces an irregular pulsing of prana. To produce a continuous inflow and outflow of prana, merely use your intent.)

3. Add a visualization, similar to the one you used in Exercise 8–B, if you wish. (But, don't visualize energy streaming into your receiving palm. Our experiments with scanning people who utilize that particular visualization revealed that it actually inhibits the amount of energy you draw in.) See a brilliant white circle superimposed on the target.

4–10. Steps 4 through 10 are the same as in Exercise 8–B.

11. Conclude by shaking your hands and spraying them with alcohol. Take a few pranic breaths and relax.

SELF-ENERGIZING YOUR OWN DEPLETED AREAS OR CHAKRAS USING THE WATER PUMP TECHNIQUE

This exercise involves performing the water pump on yourself, and it is among the most valuable techniques you will learn. Pranic Healing instructor Anthony Guidera, who travels back and forth to teach classes in Los Angeles and San Francisco, uses it as part of a routine to keep himself energized as he makes the six-hour drive between northern and southern California. He first cleanses key energy-related organs, including the spleen, liver, pancreas, kidneys, and adrenal glands, then energizes them with white prana using the water pump technique. Even with his grueling travel schedule, he says, "My body remains alert, refreshed, revitalized, and charged."

As you did with local self-scanning and self-sweeping, you can perform self-energizing using either full or partial visualization.

EXERCISE 8–D: *Self-Energizing Your Own Depleted Areas or Chakras Using the Water Pump Technique*

Perform your standard warm-up. Decide if you wish to use full or partial visualization. Perform steps 1 and 2 from Exercise 8–B, then proceed.

1. Energize this way: Put your hands in the proper position, with your energy-projecting hand 4 to 6 inches from your target area and your receiving hand palm up and slightly in front and to the side of your body. The position will be the same whether you're working on the actual area or a visualization of the area.
2. Place your awareness lightly on both palm chakras, and form your intent to draw in air and solar prana through your receiving hand and to project this prana into the target area. Example: "I now intend to draw in prana through my left hand and project it from my right hand into ____." Begin pranic breathing, and as you do, keep light awareness on the receiving and projecting palm chakras.
3. Add visualization, if you wish, imagining a brilliant white beam of light radiating from your palm into the target area. See it as a brilliant white circle superimposed on the target.

4–10. Steps 4 through 10 are the same as in Exercise 8–B, but there is no need to cut cords when you work on yourself.

11. Conclude by shaking your hands and spraying them with alcohol. Take a few pranic breaths and relax.

A Few Final Notes on Energizing

- Use intent to accelerate the absorption of energy. You can add great power to your energy work with a solid declaration of what you'd like to occur. After you send energy to a body part or chakra, silently but firmly declare, "My body (or chakra or particular body part) is absorbing the prana now."

- Don't shower or wash after you've energized. Water absorbs some of the prana intended for your deficient area or chakra, and soap—especially antibacterial or harsh soaps—wash away some prana. When you energize, not all of the prana enters the target area right away. Rather, it stays in the energy body, and the physical body assimilates it gradually. (This is also part of the reason for the healing lag time you read about in Chapter 1.) While it is waiting in the energy body, the prana is delicate. Thus you should not take a shower or bathe the energized area for at least 12 hours after a treatment. It's fine, however, to wash or bathe if all you've done is sweep the area.
- Four areas you shouldn't energize:

  The eyes. They are too delicate and can be damaged if they receive a strong dose of prana.

  The front heart chakra. It, too, can be damaged from a direct application of prana. There are some treatment sequences, though, in which you energize the heart through the back heart chakra.

  The meng mein. The *meng mein* controls the blood pressure, and energizing it can raise your blood pressure to an unhealthful level.

  The spleen chakra. This is connected to the meng mein chakra. Energizing it could stimulate the meng mein and cause the blood pressure to rise.

- Additionally, never energize a pregnant woman's navel, sex, *meng mein*, or basic chakras unless you have personal guidance from an advanced pranic healer.

ENERGIZING CHECKLIST

Self-Energizing Using the Water Pump Technique

1. Begin with standard warm-up.
2. Scan your aura, front and back, to determine the level and location of any energetic disruption.
3. Sweep and clean any congested areas—either local areas or chakras.
4. After cleaning any areas of energetic disturbance, reinforce your intent to draw in prana through your receiving hand and beam it out of your projecting hand.
5. Put your hands in the proper water pump position.
6. Place your awareness lightly on your hand chakras.
7. Begin pranic breathing, and project the prana into the area.

8. Visualize a brilliant circle of light on the target, if you wish.
9. Reinforce and drive in the prana with a clockwise rotation of your projecting hand.
10. Scan periodically as you energize.
11. Energize until: you feel a slight repulsion from the area; the area feels level with the surrounding area; you get an intuitive feeling to stop; or you reach five to seven cycles of pranic breathing (for simple problem) or 10 cycles (for more difficult problems).
12. Repeat on as many areas as are deficient.

SIX STEPS DAILY PRACTICE ROUTINE—UPDATE

As needed:

1. *Direct clearing* (Exercises 3–A and 3–B).
2. *Stretching, loosening the diaphragm* (Exercise 4–A).
3. *Hand Sensitivity Exercises 1 and 2* (Exercise 1–A and 5–A).

Daily practice:

4. *Pranic breathing* (Exercise 4–B).
5. *Scanning* (Exercises 5–B to 5–E). General and specific: yourself and other people, with and without visualization, energetic baseline, chakral baseline (Exercises 6–D and 6–E).
6. *Sweeping* (Exercises 7–B to 7–J). General and local: yourself and other people, with and without visualization, health rays, joints and body parts, chakras.
7. *Energizing* (Exercises 8–B to 8–D). Simple projection and the water pump: simple image, another person, yourself.

In the next chapter, you'll learn to enhance all of your energy manipulation work with colored pranas.

CHAPTER 9
Rainbow Power— Using Colors

"I have severe arthritis of the right knee. I had been seeing a rheumatologist regularly for treatment, which often consisted of having fluid drained from the knee and having a steroid injected into the knee to reduce inflammation. I was seriously considering going to an orthopedic surgeon to discuss a knee replacement. Dr. Robins performed two Pranic Healing treatments on the knee, which significantly decreased the pain, swelling, and inflammation.

"More important, he taught me how to apply these treatments myself. Now, whenever my knee acts up—for instance, during long trips in the car—I simply sweep the knee with light green and energize it with green and blue prana. It always makes the knee feel much better."

—BARBARA DOZIER, LOS ANGELES

When you consciously draw in and project white prana into areas of energetic disturbance in your aura, the white prana is broken down by the body's own prana into various colored pranas, much the way a prism splits white light into all the colors of the spectrum. Each color of prana produces a particular healing effect, in a particular way and at a particular pace. The body assimilates the colored pranas that it needs from the white prana, based on what healing effects are required to remedy the problem. Thus, when you use white prana for healing, not all the energy you draw in and project is utilized to heal the problem; some is siphoned off into your body's general energy reservoir. This isn't wasteful; after all, you still keep all the prana within your energy body. It's just not as efficient a healing effort as it could be.

Through the use of colored pranas, though, you can produce quicker, more efficient healing. By applying only those colors of pranas that produce the specific healing effect that a particular health problem requires, your energy will be more focused and concentrated, which is especially important when addressing difficult or complex health problems.

THE BASICS OF USING COLORED PRANAS

There are seven single-colored pranas: red, yellow, orange, blue, green, violet, and electric violet. There are also dual-colored pranas that combine two colors for a specific potent effect—for example, green-blue prana. (*Note:* Among single-colored pranas, there is also gold prana, and there are other dual-colored pranas. But gold prana and most dual-colored pranas are used only by advanced healers in specific situations. We won't cover them in this book. Nevertheless, the colored pranas you learn here are extremely powerful and effective for healing.) Each color of prana has a specific rate of vibration and a grade of refinement, both of which are determined by the size of the particles that make up the prana. The vibration rate and grade of refinement, in turn, determine the prana's healing application (see Table 9–1). In general, low-vibration pranas are used for heavy-duty healing such as repairing torn tissues and broken bones, while high-vibration pranas are used for more sensitive healing efforts, such as energizing nerve tissue.

The prana with the lowest rate of vibration and refinement, and with the largest particles, is red. The prana with the highest rate of vibration and refinement, and with the tiniest particles, is electric violet. Blue and green prana are in the middle. Here's how to think of the differences in vibrational rate in relation to the size of the energy particles that make up the prana: Take a shirt button, a golf ball, and a softball. Put them in an empty shoe box one at a time and shake vigorously. Which moves around the fastest and easiest? Which is the slowest? The shirt button is comparable to violet prana, the golf ball to green and blue, and the softball to red.

SWEEPING AND ENERGIZING WITH COLORED PRANAS

Sweeping and energizing with colored pranas builds on the techniques you've already learned. When you swept your energetic anatomy, you used beams of white light to scrape away the dirty energy. When you energized, you projected white prana by drawing it in through the palm chakra of one hand and emitting it through the palm chakra of the other. You use the exact same principles with colored pranas; you just use the different source chakras as "filters" or "lenses" to transform the white prana into the color prana you need. For instance, when you sweep with a particular color, you simply put your awareness on the source chakra, form your intent to draw in prana through that source chakra, and then visualize the desired color beaming from your fingertips and sweeping away the dirty energy.

Table 9-I	COLORED PRANAS AND THEIR CHARACTERISTICS			
Colored Prana	Primary Healing Characteristic	Application	Examples of Use	Source Chakra
Red	Warm	Strengthening, stimulating, activating, dilating, expanding, growing	Energizing deficient lower chakras, boosting overall energy, energizing nondelicate organs, increasing blood flow	Basic
Yellow	Cementing	Hardening, initiating, triggering	Promoting tissue growth, wound repair	Basic
Orange	Expelling (through splitting or exploding)	Rapid, heavy-duty cleansing; eliminating quickly and dramatically	Relieving constipation, removing heavy congestion from nondelicate areas	Basic
Green	Breaking down (chopping)	Cleansing, dissolving, decongesting, loosening, disinfecting	Cleansing and energizing any area, delicate or nondelicate	Throat
Blue	Cooling	Soothing, localizing, inhibiting	Stopping or reducing bleeding, pain relief, stabilizing prana	Throat
Green-blue	Chopping/cooling	Strong disinfecting, soothing	Relieving pain	Throat
Violet	All properties	Cleansing, disinfecting, regenerating; magnifying effect on other pranas	Cleansing and energizing any area, delicate or nondelicate	Crown
Electric violet (divine spiritual energy)	All properties	Like violet, but even more powerful	Cleansing and energizing any area; emotional disturbances	Crown

To energize with a particular color, you put your awareness on the source chakra, form your intent to draw in prana through that source chakra, and then visualize the desired color beaming from the palm chakra of your projecting hand into the deficient area.

Colors Produce Specific Energetic Effects

"One evening when I was on call in the emergency room, a chemotherapy patient came in with severe diarrhea and dehydration. The standard remedy is to insert an IV so we can administer fluids. But chemotherapy patients often have very poor veins—either too small or collapsed from dehydration. Six different nurses tried to put in an IV line, but no one could find a good enough vein. At this point, a surgeon was called in to do a 'cut-down,' which entails cutting the skin over the ankle to find and utilize the saphenous vein for the IV. As the surgeon was responding from another part of the hospital, I remembered that red prana causes 'dilation.' I energized this patient's arm with red prana for about 90 seconds, and then all of a sudden a large vein popped up, seemingly from nowhere. I was able to place the IV needle, and the minor surgery was canceled. Needless to say, the patient was delighted."

—*Eric B. Robins, M.D.*

Here's how one Pranic Healing instructor, Daniel O'Hara, used his knowledge of colored prana to save his vacation and prevent a trip to an emergency room:

"*At a sushi bar while on vacation in Las Vegas with some friends, I asked the sushi chef, who had been gruff with us all evening, for some really hot and spicy food. The chef quickly placed a large piece of sushi with a quail egg on top of it in front of me. After putting the whole piece into my mouth, I immediately realized what he had done: It was a clump of pure wasabi, the hot green sushi mustard, about four times the size that usually comes with an entire plate of sushi. Not wanting to give this guy the pleasure of seeing me sweat—literally—I excused myself to the rest room. My face was red, and my stomach felt like it was full of molten lava. I kept sweeping my stomach and my solar plexus and navel chakras with green and violet, which immediately minimized the pain. I then energized the area with green, violet, blue, and white pranas. Within 5 minutes the discomfort was gone, and I returned to the table to join my friends. Without Pranic Healing, I'm sure we would have had to take a trip to the local hospital.*"

As detailed in Table 9–1, you use your *basic chakra* to project in the lower vibrational colors: red, yellow and orange. The basic draws in very physical, low-vibrational energy because it is close to the earth and also because it is through the basic chakra that you root yourself energetically to the earth. Prana drawn in through the basic is primarily ground prana with some air prana.

You use your *throat chakra* to project middle-vibrational colors: green, blue, and the dual-colored green-blue. The throat draws in slightly more refined prana because it is not as close to the ground; prana drawn in through the throat chakra is primarily air prana.

You use your *crown* to project violet and electric violet prana. Since the crown can produce color from any chakra, you may also use the crown as your source chakra when you use dual-colored pranas. The crown also draws in the most refined energy of your source chakras: air prana and divine spiritual energy.

GENERAL GUIDELINES FOR SAFE AND PROPER USAGE OF COLORED PRANAS

Colored pranas are more powerful than white prana, and you need to be more careful with them. But if you follow these basic guidelines, you should encounter no problems:

1. *Always project a pastel ring of color with a white center rather than a solid shade.* The preferred projection is a bright white disk with a pastel ring of the colored prana you wish to project around its circumference. Dark-colored pranas are very strong energy, are difficult for any healer to control, especially a beginner, and can damage delicate areas. Dark-colored pranas should be used only by very experienced healers in select instances.

   Grandmaster Choa Kok Sui's experiments revealed that light-colored rings of prana produce quicker, more effective healings. By using bright white prana in the center of the projected ring, you allow the body to absorb minute amounts of any other colors of prana it may need for healing.

2. *Always project a color that is one shade lighter than you need.* Grandmaster Choa's research revealed that most people, particularly beginners, project a shade much darker than they think they're projecting, mainly because dark colors are easier to visualize than pastels. To avoid projecting prana that is too dark, review Table 9–II and then make a conscious effort, with your intent, to project pastels.

   For instance, you will see in Chapter 13 that part of the energetic remedy for relieving menstrual cramps is to project light whitish-green and light whitish-orange prana into the sex chakra. In the "early days" of Pranic Healing, while these techniques were still being refined, Grandmaster Choa Kok Sui found that people who projected solid or darker colors would relieve the discomfort—often quickly. But the women invariably got diarrhea after the healing because the darker colors projected into the lower abdomen, particularly orange, would cause loose bowel movements.

Table 9-II PROJECTING COLORED PRANA	
If you want to project this color . . .	**Use your intent to focus on and visualize a bright white disk with this color around the circumference**
Red	Light pink
Orange	Light peach
Yellow	Light yellow, almost beige
Green	Light apple green
Blue	Sky blue or baby blue
Violet	Light lavender
Electric violet	Blinding white, or a lightning bolt with faint lavender at the edges

3. *Colored prana cautions:*
   - Don't mix violet or electric violet with red, yellow, or orange. Both violet and electric violet have dramatic magnifying effects, and when mixed with these already-potent pranas, it is too strong.
   - Don't use orange on the abdomen if you have diarrhea. It worsens the problem.
   - Don't use colors on children or infants. Colored pranas are too strong for them.
   - Don't use red or orange on the sex chakra to treat venereal disease, prostate cancer, or ovarian cancer. It spreads the problem.
   - Don't use colors on pregnant women. They could damage the fetus.

- Don't mix red and yellow. Dirty red and dirty yellow are the energy colors of cancer. The cancer cells are rapidly growing (red) and hardening (yellow).

4. *Always follow the rules for using colors on delicate areas.* Certain parts of your body are delicate and can be damaged by stronger prana. These delicate areas include the head (because of the brain), the heart (because of the heart and lungs), and the spleen (because the spleen is like a pump, sending everything through the body via the blood). We also recommend that beginners treat the throat and solar plexus chakras as delicate, because of their proximity to the head and heart, respectively. *Never use orange to sweep or red to energize delicate areas!* Treat such areas only with milder pranas, such as white, green, blue, and violet. If you're unsure whether the area is delicate, or you feel you don't have sufficient control over colored prana, treat the area as if it were delicate.

PROGRESSIVE USE OF COLORS EXERCISES

From this point forward, we omit formal references to practicing on other people. It's understood that you may continue to practice on other people as you wish or are able.

Here is the sequence of progressive use of colors exercises:

1. Visualization practice with colors
2. Self-sweeping with colors
3. Self-energizing with colors
4. Testing pranic flow of water pump technique

Follow the same step-by-step sequence as in learning all the energy-manipulation skills. Even though you use visualization more when using colored pranas, intent and proper technique are still more important to success than visualization. If you can visualize well, it makes your healing with colors more effective. But don't be concerned if your visualization skills aren't where you want them to be just yet. Continue your practice.

As you practice with colored prana, you may find that each has a different feel. Long-time Pranic Healing practitioner Arnon Davidovici reports that when he projects red, his hand immediately warms up; with orange, his hand tingles; with yellow, the energy feels harder and heavier; with green, the energy feels smooth and flowing; with blue, it feels like cool air is brushing against his hand; with orange, his hand tingles; with violet, his hand feels light, as if it's floating; and with electric violet, his hand floats and tingles.

VISUALIZATION PRACTICE WITH COLORS

While the exercises in this chapter focus on projecting prana, or energizing, the same principles apply to sweeping with colors. With both sweeping and energizing, begin by keeping your awareness on the source chakra. When you sweep, visualize the colored beams extending from your fingertips; when you energize, visualize the prana emitting from your palm chakra.

EXERCISE 9–A: *Visualization Practice with Colors—Single Colors*

You can stand or sit for the exercise. Perform your standard warm-up.

1. Establish a target for your visualization. Put a sheet of unlined white paper or cardboard on the ground in front of you or on the wall. If your wall is white or light-colored, that will work. The target should be 1 to 2 feet in front of you.

2. Tap your source chakra lightly twice with your nonprojecting hand to focus your attention and establish your intent. Begin with projecting green, so tap your throat chakra (Figure 9–1).

3. Perform three more cycles of pranic breathing.

4. Put your projecting hand in the proper position facing the target. Keep your other hand at your side, or on your hip or in your pocket. Continue pranic breathing, and as you do, keep light awareness on the source and projecting chakras.

5. From this point forward, use a short-cut visualization. Just see the pastel ring superimposed on your target, rather than tracing the beam of prana from your projecting palm to the target as you did with the flashlight in Exercise 8–A. That exercise helps you learn what a visualization looks like, and it is good practice. But in the reality of healing, all you need do is visualize the ring on your target. Project a pastel ring of green prana with a bright white center about 6 inches in diameter onto your target for four cycles of pranic breathing (Figure 9–2).

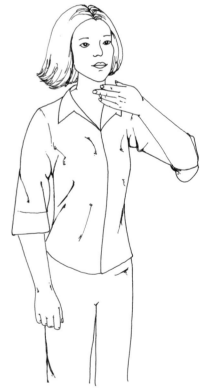

FIGURE 9–1

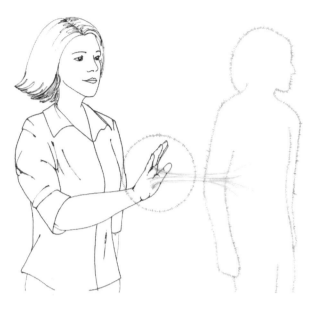

FIGURE 9–2

6. As you breathe and project, keep your awareness on your source and projecting chakras more than on your breathing. Utilize the short-cut visualization, seeing just the ring on your target rather than following the beam from your projecting hand. If at any time you need to refocus your intent, simply declare to yourself that you intend to project light green prana onto this target.

7. Rest and relax. Shake your hands. Then repeat the exercise three more times.

8. Next, project blue. Begin by flicking your hands downward a few times. (Flicking your hands between colors is important. It's like a painter washing his brush before using another color.) Then follow steps 2 through 7 for blue.

9. Using the same steps, project red and yellow from your basic, and violet and electric violet from your crown. Take your time and, as with the flashlight exercise, have fun with it. One of the keys to successful visualization is to really use your imagination. Be creative and have fun when you visualize.

EXERCISE 9–B: *Visualization Practice with Colors—Dual Colors (Green-Blue)*

In dual-colored pranas, the first color in the pair is the lesser of the two colors, meaning there is less green and more blue in green-blue. The lesser color is also the inside ring. The center is bright white.

There are two ways to project dual-colored prana: Visualize the inner ring first, then surround it with the outer ring, or visualize both rings simultaneously. But most beginners find it simpler to project the colors one at a time. Experiment and see which is easier for you.

If you continue with Exercise 9–B immediately after Exercise 9–A, there is no need to go through the warm-up steps again. But if you begin your practice with Exercise 9–B, use the standard warm-up and steps 1 through 4 from Exercise 9–A, then proceed.

1. Begin pranic breathing, and as you do, keep light awareness on the source and projecting chakras. Project a pastel ring of green-blue prana about 6 inches in diameter onto your target for four cycles of pranic breathing. Either visualize them in sequence, with green as the inside ring and then blue outside the green, or visualize both at the same time.

2. Keep your awareness on your source and projecting chakras more than on your breathing. By this time, pranic breathing should be second nature to you. Utilize the short-cut visualization in Exercise 9–A, seeing just the ring on your target rather than following the beam from your projecting hand. If at any time you need to refocus your intent, simply declare to yourself that you intend to project green-blue prana onto this target.

3. Rest and relax. Shake your hands. Then repeat the exercise three more times.

SELF-SWEEPING WITH COLORS

In general self-sweeping with colors, you use green prana instead of white. If you have the time or need, you may add a second round of general self-sweeping with violet prana.

In local self-sweeping with colors, you use green and orange pranas alternately on non-delicate areas and chakras, and green and violet alternately on delicate areas and chakras. Sweeping "alternately" means to sweep with two sets of five sweeps with the first color (e.g., green), then with two sets of five sweeps of the second color (e.g., green or violet).

EXERCISE 9–C: *General Self-Sweeping with Colors*

You may sit or stand for this exercise. Perform your standard warm-up.

1. Establish a quick energetic baseline for yourself (Exercise 6–D). Note the relative shape and strength of your aura, as well as any areas of congestion or depletion.

2. If necessary, reestablish your intent by silently declaring to yourself that you intend to sweep and clean away the dirty prana from your energy body.

3. Using your preferred visualization technique, imagine yourself about 2 to 3 feet in front of you. Remember that you can increase identification with your visualization by saying your name three times.

4. Tap your throat chakra, and form an intent to draw in prana through the throat chakra and project green beams through your fingertips.

5. With your hands in the slightly cupped general sweeping position, aim your fingers slightly above the head of your visualized body.

6. Imagine the beams of green light emanating from your fingers and penetrating an inch or two into your visualized body. Remember that depth in scanning is determined by intent.

7. Follow the general self-sweeping sequence (Exercise 7–F). Begin pranic breathing, but keep your awareness more on your sweeping movement than on your pranic breathing or a visualization of the beams. By this time, pranic breathing should be second nature to you.

8. After sweeping the front of your visualized figure, turn it around and sweep the back.

9. If you have the time and need, perform a second set of 10 sweeps—five on the front and five on the back—with violet. Flick your hands downward a few times because you're changing colors. Tap your crown chakra and form a clear intent to sweep with violet. Visualize light violet beams emitting from your fingertips, and begin your sweeping passes.

10. After you complete your sweeping, rescan your aura. Note if it seems more balanced now. Note also if you feel lighter, more relaxed, or more refreshed.

11. Conclude the exercise by shaking your hands and spraying them with alcohol again. Take a few pranic breaths and relax.

Many people find that one 10-sweep routine with green is sufficient for general cleansing. A second 10-sweep pass with violet, however, is very beneficial if you have time. If you are pressed for time, or you want a short-cut alternate with violet, you can sweep with green for 10 passes, then just sweep your front and back center lines with violet.

EXERCISE 9–D: *Local Self-Sweeping with Colors*

You may sit or stand for this exercise.

You'll use the front solar plexus as your target. Decide whether to use visualization. Since you're just beginning, we'll consider this to be a delicate area, which means you will sweep with green and violet alternately.

Perform your standard warm-up.

1. Scan your front solar plexus chakra for all three dimensions, noting any congestion or depletion.

2. Tap your throat chakra, and form an intent to draw in prana through the throat chakra and project green beams through your fingertips. Begin pranic breathing, but keep your awareness more on your sweeping movement than on your pranic breathing or a visualization of the beams. By this time pranic breathing should be second nature to you.

3. With your dominant hand in the slightly cupped sweeping position, turn it backward so that your fingers are pointing at your front solar plexus chakra from 4 to 6 inches away (Figure 9–3). If you're using full visualization, imagine your fingertips 4 to 6 inches away from your imagined body. Begin sweeping with a tight counterclockwise motion of the wrist, one second per revolution. (Remember how to determine counterclockwise: Imagine a watch with its face outward lying on your target.) Visualize light-green beams extending from your fingers and penetrating several inches into the skin to scrape out grayish-brown dirty energy.

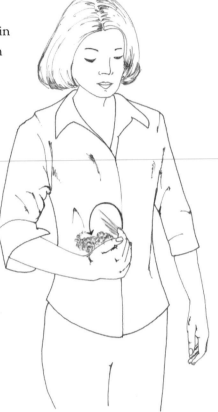

FIGURE 9–3

4. After five revolutions, pull your hand down and away and flick it into the salt water. Perform another set of five counterclockwise sweeps with green. Spray your hand with alcohol.

5. Flick your hand downward a few times, because you're going to change colors. Tap your crown chakra, and form a clear intent to sweep with violet. Visualize light violet beams emitting from your fingertips.

6. Resume your chakra sweeping hand posture, and perform two sets of counterclockwise sweeping passes on your front solar plexus with light violet. After completing two sets, spray your hand with alcohol, and flick your hands downward.

7. Then tap your throat again, form an intent to sweep with green prana, and perform two sets of five counterclockwise sweeps with green. Spray with alcohol, then flick your hand downward.

8. Tap your crown, form an intent to sweep with violet prana, and perform two sets of five counterclockwise sweeps with green. Spray with alcohol, then flick your hand downward.

9. Continue sweeping alternately with green and violet until you've completed 60 total sweeps of your front solar plexus chakra.

10. Rescan your front solar plexus chakra. If it's still congested, continue with your sweeping until scanning reveals that the congestion is gone.

11. Conclude the exercise by shaking your hands and spraying them with alcohol again. Take a few pranic breaths, and relax.

For a local area or joint, apply these principles to the dog-paddle sweeping method (Exercise 7–I). Sweep alternately with green then violet if the area is delicate and with green then orange if the area is nondelicate. Or, if you wish, stick with green and violet for all local sweeping. Remember to flick your fingers and tap your source chakra to establish your intent before changing colors.

EXERCISE 9–E: *Advanced General Self-Sweeping with Colors*

This exercise adds energizing to your general cleansing routine. It takes more practice, but is a very effective cleansing exercise. (There is also an advanced local self-sweeping routine, but it is beyond the scope of this book.)

You may sit or stand. Perform your standard warm-up. Begin with steps 1 through 3 from Exercise 9–C, then proceed.

1. Tap your throat chakra, and form an intent to draw in prana through the throat chakra and project green beams through *both* hands. Begin pranic breathing, but keep your awareness more on sweeping than on your pranic breathing.

2. Turn your visualization sideways, and position your hands so that one palm chakra is lined up with the front solar plexus chakra and the other is lined up with the back solar plexus chakra (Figure 9–4).

3. Fill your entire visualized body with light green prana. Let it flow through your hands into the solar plexus chakras. You may want to visualize your body as hollow, with the green prana flowing into your feet first, then filling up your entire body. All your muscles, bones, skin, organs, hair should be light green. Picture yourself slightly glowing. After your body is filled, stabilize both the front and back solar plexus chakras with light blue.

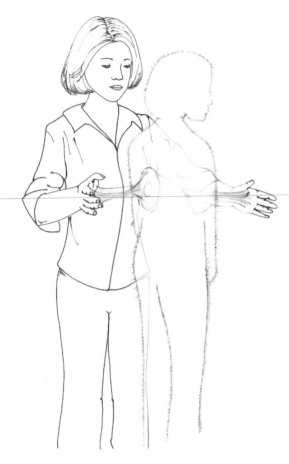

FIGURE 9–4

4. Now break contact with the visualization for a moment to allow the green prana to "cook." This will loosen up the dirty energy the way pretreating loosens up a stain on a shirt before you throw it into the laundry.

5. After a few moments, go back and perform regular general sweeping on your visualization, both front and back, with light green.

6. After you complete your sweeping, rescan your aura. See if it seems more balanced now. Note also if you feel lighter, more relaxed, or more refreshed.

7. Conclude the exercise by shaking your hands and spraying them with alcohol again. Relax.

This is a quicker, more thorough way to clean your energy body than general self-sweeping, but it does require more practice. Most students, after they master the advanced method, seldom go back to regular general self-sweeping.

SELF-ENERGIZING WITH COLORS

To self-energize with colors, you use the water pump method to draw the color prana you need through your various source chakras. It's the same visualization practice as in Exercises 9–A and 9–B, but with a live target rather than the wall or a piece of paper.

Your first exercise in this section is an actual remedy, similar to the step-by-step remedies in Chapter 13: Its purpose is to relieve stress.

EXERCISE 9–F: *Self-Energizing with Colors—Stress Relief*

Preparation is the same as for Exercise 9–C. Decide whether you'll use full or partial visualization.

1. Establish a quick energetic baseline (Exercise 6–D). Note the relative shape and strength of your aura, as well as any areas of congestion or depletion. Note in particular the condition of the chakras on which you will work in this routine: the front and back solar plexus chakras, the *meng mein*, the throat chakra, and the *ajna*. Because the solar plexus chakras control our emotions, they are frequently out of balance energetically during stressful periods. The *meng mein* controls your blood pressure and other key physiological functions involved in the body's reaction to stress. The throat chakra is a center of creativity and sensitivity that frequently is affected by stress. And the *ajna* is the seat of persistent negative thoughts, which frequently accompany stress.
2. Perform general self-sweeping with colors, using either the 10-sweep method, Exercise 9–D, or the advanced method, Exercise 9–E.
3. Scan the front solar plexus chakra to determine its energetic level. Sweep and clean the front solar plexus chakra alternately with light green and light violet. "Alternately" means to sweep with two sets of five sweeps with one color (total of 10), and then sweep with two sets of five sweeps with the other color (total of 10). Sweep with 60 total sweeps or until you feel a reduction in congestion.
4. Energize the front solar plexus chakra with light green. Tap your source chakra, your throat, lightly with your nonprojecting hand twice to focus your attention and establish your intent. If you are using visualization, place your projecting hand 4 to 6 inches away from your target. If you're working on yourself, turn it back toward you so that your hand is 4 to 6 inches from your front solar plexus chakra (Figure 9–5). Project a pastel ring of light green with a bright white center about 4 inches in diameter onto your front solar plexus chakra for five cycles of pranic breathing. Keep your awareness

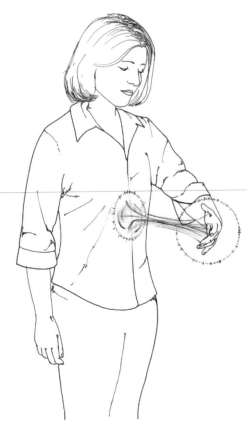

FIGURE 9–5

on your source and projecting chakras more than your breathing. Utilize the short-cut visualization (Exercise 9–A), seeing just the ring on your target rather than following the beam from your projecting hand. You may drive in the prana with a slight clockwise rotation of your hand.

5. When you are finished, pull your hand away from the front solar plexus chakra, and shake your fingers downward a few times.

6. Energize the front solar plexus chakra with light violet. Use the same routine as you used for projecting light green, but use the crown as your source chakra.

7. When you are finished, pull your hand away from the front solar plexus chakra and shake your fingers downward a few times. Stabilize the front solar plexus chakra with light blue. You should be quite relaxed.

8. Sweep and clean the back solar plexus chakra alternately with light green and light violet for a total of 60 sweeps or until you feel a reduction in congestion.

9. Energize the back solar plexus chakra with light green, light blue, then light violet. Stabilize with light blue.

10. Sweep and clean the *meng mein* alternately with light green and light violet for a total of 60 sweeps or until you feel a reduction in congestion. Stabilize with light blue.

11. Sweep and clean the throat chakra alternately with light green and light violet for a total of 60 sweeps or until you feel a reduction in congestion.

12. Energize it lightly with light violet only. You energize lightly by using less will than you do normally and by easing up on your visualization. Your intent will determine your degree of energizing. Stabilize with light blue.

13. Next, sweep and clean the *ajna* alternately with light green and light violet for a total of 60 sweeps or until you feel a reduction in congestion.

14. Energize it lightly with light violet only. Stabilize with light blue.

15. Rescan your aura and the specific areas you worked on. If you've over-energized, sweep away the excess congestion.

16. Conclude by shaking your hands and spraying them with alcohol. Take a few pranic breaths and relax.

TESTING YOUR PRANIC FLOW DURING THE WATER PUMP TECHNIQUE

Positive feedback helps your progress. If you are fortunate enough to be learning this material with someone else, here is a two-person exercise that will easily and quickly enable you to learn whether, when you project energy, you're drawing prana in through your chakras from outside your body or using your own supply.

EXERCISE 9–G: *Testing Your Pranic Flow*

Stand for this exercise. Have your partner stand behind you at an angle that will enable him to scan your basic chakra. We use the basic chakra because it's easy for a partner to scan. The exercise steps are written as if you were projecting prana and your partner were testing you, but you should test each other.

Both of you should perform a standard warm-up.

1. Establish a target for your visualization: a sheet of paper, the wall, or just visualize your target. The target should be 1 to 2 feet in front of you.

2. Have your partner scan your basic chakra before you begin projecting prana, so you know its size and strength before starting the test.

3. Tap your source chakra, the basic, which is located at the base of the spine, twice lightly with your nonprojecting hand to focus your attention and help establish your intent.

4. Raise your projecting hand toward the target in the proper posture. Just keep your other hand at your side, or on your hip or in your pocket.

5. Project a pastel ring of red prana with a bright white center 4 to 6 inches in diameter onto your target for four cycles of pranic breathing. Keep your awareness lightly on the source and projecting chakra.

6. As you project, have your partner scan your basic chakra again, both its width and its depth. If you are drawing prana in through the basic, your partner should feel the basic chakra expand and strengthen. If you are drawing prana from your own body, your basic chakra will remain unchanged, or it may shrink.

If you aren't drawing in prana through your basic, just relax and continue your practice. Reinforcing your intent periodically to draw in prana as you energize is all it takes to get the flow of prana started.

A Few Final Notes on Working with Colored Pranas

- Electric violet is best visualized as a circle of pure blinding white light, or lightning with faint lavender edges. Here are several ways to do that: Think of the fuse on a firecracker, the tip of a Fourth of July sparkler, or sunlight reflecting off newly fallen snow. All of these produce a brilliant white flash of light.

- Here are some advanced visualization drills: Eliminate your practice target. Rather than projecting your visualization onto a wall or sheet of paper, visualize a target in the air in front of you, and then see your pastel ring on that. Also, adjust the size of your colored prana ring, using your intent and visualization ability.

- After you become more comfortable with establishing your intent, you no longer need to tap your source chakra. Just mentally put your intent there without physically touching it.

- If, as you scan, you encounter a local area of tough congestion that resists regular local sweeping, poke it with green prana. Form a clear intent to break up the congestion, be aware of your throat chakra, and visualize green beams coming from the first two fingers of your scanning hand. Poke in sets of ten. Then sweep away with light green. This works particularly well for arthritic joints.

USING COLORED PRANAS CHECKLIST

(*Note*: Use the standard warm-up before all practice sessions.)

General Self-Sweeping with Colored Pranas

1. Establish your energetic baseline; or scan your aura, front and back, to determine the level and possible location of energetic disruption.
2. Tap your throat chakra to place awareness there, and focus your intent on sweeping with light green.
3. Visualize your hands as large green paddles or with light green beams emerging from fingertips.
4. Do a first head-to-toe sweep down the center line, using visualization if you wish.
5. Flick dirty prana into salt water.
6. Separate your hands by one and a half hand-widths for a second head-to-toe sweep.
7. Flick dirty prana into salt water.
8. Spray your hands with alcohol.
9. Continue sweeping, maintaining a slight overlap as you move your hands outward by one and a half hand-widths each time.
10. Spray your hands with alcohol after every two passes.
11. On the fifth and final sweep, with your hands slightly outstretched, trace the outline of your body.
12. Repeat on back.
13. Tap your crown chakra to place awareness there, and focus your intent on sweeping with light violet.
14. Visualize your hands as large violet paddles or with light violet beams emerging from the fingertips.
15. Repeat steps 4 through 12 with violet.

Local Self-Sweeping of Joint or Small Body Area with Colored Pranas

1. Scan the target to determine the level and location of the energetic congestion.
2. Tap your source chakra to place awareness there, and focus your intent on sweeping with whatever color prana you need.
3. Visualize your hands with colored beams emerging from the fingertips.

4. Do a first set of five to ten dog paddles, using visualization if you wish.
5. Flick dirty prana into salt water.
6. Do a second set of five to ten dog paddles.
7. Flick dirty prana into salt water.
8. Spray your hand with alcohol.
9. Continue sweeping and then scanning periodically until scanning reveals that the area is clean.
10. Spray your hand with alcohol after every two passes.

Local Self-Sweeping of Chakra with Colors

1. Scan the target chakra to determine the level of energy.
2. Tap your source chakra to place awareness there, and focus your intent on sweeping with whatever color prana you need.
3. Visualize your hands with colored beams emerging from the fingertips.
4. Do a first set of five counterclockwise sweeps, using visualization if you wish.
5. Flick dirty prana into salt water.
6. Do a second set of five counterclockwise sweeps.
7. Flick dirty prana into salt water.
8. Spray your hand with alcohol.
9. Continue sweeping and then scanning periodically until scanning reveals that the area is clean.
10. Spray your hand with alcohol after every two passes.

Self-Energizing Using the Water Pump Technique with Colored Pranas

1. Establish the energetic baseline; or scan your aura, front and back, to determine the level and possible location of energetic disruption.
2. Sweep and clean any congested areas—either local areas or chakras.
3. When you find a local area of energetic disturbance, clean it, then reinforce your intent to draw in prana through the appropriate source chakra according to the color you need, and beam it out of your projecting hand.
4. Put your hands in the proper water pump position.
5. Place your awareness lightly on your source and projecting chakras.

6. Begin pranic breathing, and project the prana into the area—5 to 7 cycles for a simple ailment; 10 or more cycles for a more difficult problem.

7. Visualize a bright white circle of light on the target surrounded by a pastel ring of your selected color.

8. Reinforce and drive the prana in with a slight clockwise rotation of your projecting hand.

9. Remember to scan periodically as you energize.

10. Energize until: you feel a slight repulsion from the area; the area feels level with the surrounding area; you get an intuitive feeling to stop; or you reach 5 to 7 cycles of pranic breathing (for simple problem) or 10 cycles (for a more difficult problem).

11. Repeat on as many areas as are deficient.

SIX STEPS DAILY PRACTICE ROUTINE—UPDATE

As needed:

1. *Direct clearing techniques* (Exercises 3–A and 3–B).
2. *Stretching, loosening the diaphragm exercises* (Exercise 4–A).
3. *Hand Sensitivity Exercises 1 and 2* (Exercises 1–A and 5–A).

Daily practice:

4. *Pranic breathing* (Exercise 4–B).
5. *Scanning* (Exercises 5–B to 5–E). General and specific: yourself and other people, with and without visualization, energetic baseline, chakral baseline.
6. *Visualization practice with colors* (Exercises 9–A and 9–B). Project single and dual colors onto a wall or sheet of paper; into generic human figure.
7. *General sweeping with colors* (Exercises 9–C to 9–E). General and local: yourself and other people, with and without visualization, health rays, joints and body parts, chakras; advanced general sweeping.
8. *Energizing with colors* (Exercuse 9–F). Another person, yourself.
9. *Testing pranic flow* (Exercise 9–G). Try this a couple times if you're practicing with a friend, then you needn't do it again.

An excellent all-purpose exercise that you could use in place of a set practice routine is the stress-relief exercise (Exercise 9–F). Perform it on yourself twice a week. It incorporates scanning, sweeping, and energizing, and it delivers great benefit to you.

You've now learned all the fundamentals of effective energy healing. In the next chapter, you'll learn the fourth of the six steps to self-healing, *energetic hygiene*, a practice, unique to pranic healing, of making healthful choices to maintain a high energy level.

CHAPTER 10

Keep It Clean—
The Importance of
Energetic Hygiene

"At the outset of one of my introductory classes for Pranic Healing, I asked the students, as I typically do, a little bit about their lives, the nature of their work, and what brought them to this class. One young woman stated that she was a social worker for two adult substance-abuse programs, and that she had just been served with divorce papers that day. She looked tired, and her posture was hunched over. I felt that 'cutting her cords'—the thin strands of prana that connect us energetically to anything in our lives that evokes a strong emotion in us—could help, so I asked her if she would be willing to try an experiment. She agreed, so I gathered and cut all the cords that had attached her to her work and personal issues. She began crying immediately and said she felt so much relief. She admitted that, in addition to her work and personal stresses, she was also bulimic. We cut the cord to that issue. Several days later she came to class and told everyone that she had gone five days without a bulimic episode and that her life had already changed and work was less stressful."

—SHEEVAUN O'CONNOR, PRANIC HEALING INSTRUCTOR,
HUNTINGTON BEACH, CALIFORNIA

It takes work to keep your energy body clean. Because you are part of a dynamic bio-energetic system, you encounter both the prana that sustains life and the contaminants that diminish that prana. Fresh prana is added to the system from the sun, the ultimate source, but even as living things absorb and use this fresh prana—your energy body "breathes" just as your respiratory system does—they also discharge dirty prana back into the system. Some of this expelled dirty prana is broken down naturally, but a portion stays in the air and the ground as residual contamination. Thus, we are vulnerable to *environ-*

mental contamination, or absorbing dirty prana from the air we breathe, the food and water we consume, and the places where we live and work.

Additionally, as we move through this bioenergetic system, we often find ourselves unavoidably in close proximity to other people who are not always positive, and in situations that evoke negative responses in us. We live and work with people who are angry, intentionally hurtful, or otherwise emotionally destructive. Many personal, societal, and familial influences cause us to have or hold on to stresses, worries, negative emotions, and limiting beliefs. Negativity of any kind—whether the source is work or home, general life circumstances, the actions or words of another person, or simply our own unresolved anxieties—diminishes and contaminates our personal energy supply and creates *emotional contamination*.

Although we live in an energetically dirty world and can't completely eliminate contamination, we can mitigate it through *energetic hygiene*, the practice of keeping your personal energy tank as clean and full as possible. Energetic hygiene is the fourth of the six steps to self-healing.

THE KEYS TO ENERGETIC HYGIENE

When you practice energetic hygiene diligently, your energy body becomes more refined; the particles of prana that make up your energy aura become cleaner and smaller. They also vibrate at a higher frequency. A refined energy body is able to absorb more prana of all frequencies. This quality of refinement is compounded—as you practice good energetic hygiene, you can absorb more prana, which in turn makes your energy body even more refined, which then enables you to take in even more prana, and so on. A refined energy body is also stronger energetically, which enables you to resist ailments more effectively and rebound more quickly if you do get sick.

There are five keys to energetic hygiene: *emotional regulation*, *proper diet*, *physical exercise*, *clean environment*, and a final special key, the frequent *use of salt*, in all its cleansing applications.

EMOTIONAL REGULATION

Emotional regulation is control over the toxic effect of negative emotions and limiting beliefs, whether they originate within us (self-contamination) or within other people who then direct that negativity toward us (contamination from others). In Chapter 2, you learned several direct clearing techniques to mitigate emotional self-contamination: the practices of self-awareness and higher-level thinking. You also know how to use the indirect clearing ability of pranic breathing and how to clean emotionally caused dirty energy from your aura with self-sweeping. We'll teach another indirect clearing technique, meditation, in Chapter 11.

In this chapter, we present two techniques to mitigate emotional contamination from other people who are negative, angry, fearful, or destructive and who spread that emotional and energetic toxicity to people around them: a special application of cord cutting, and a method of closing your aura to negativity.

Before you go to the emotional regulation techniques, please try this two-person experiment that demonstrates the harmful health effect of negative emotions and the healing power of positive emotions.

EXERCISE 10–A: *The Effects of Negative and Positive Emotions on Energy Level and Health*

Both you and your subject should stand. You should be behind your subject at a distance that will enable you to scan his aura comfortably. Both of you should perform a standard warm-up.

1. Scan your subject's aura at several points to establish a quick energetic baseline. Note its depth and strength.
2. Instruct your subject to conjure up a strong negative emotion, such as anger, by remembering or imagining he's in a situation that provoked him. Have him associate fully with the feeling by placing himself right there in the circumstances. Maybe he imagines himself driving and getting cut off, or being kept on hold on the phone.
3. Ask him to add physical postural elements that express his anger: a scowl, a frown, a hunching of the shoulders, crossing the arms aggressively. He may even hear himself cursing.
4. While your subject is at the peak of his angry state, rescan him. You will find a decrease in the depth and strength of his aura at every point. You may also find the front or back solar plexus chakras to be depleted or congested, depending upon the person.
5. Call the subject out of his negative state, and have him walk around for a minute or two and perform several cycles of pranic breathing to relax.

6. Then have your subject conjure up a strong positive emotion, such as love, by imagining or remembering a situation of love. He may imagine himself with a loved one or relive a particularly happy moment from his life. Have him associate fully with the feeling and show it in his more relaxed face and body. Have him hear himself saying loving words and feeling them.

7. At the peak of this positive emotional state, scan your subject. You will find an increase in the depth and strength of the aura. You may also find the front and back heart and solar plexus chakras substantially strengthened.

Perform this experiment with different people and different emotions (fear, anger, anxiety, love, joy, happiness, and so on). People invariably find that negative emotions reduce or congest their energy, while positive emotions increase and expand their energy. This simple, profound exercise demonstrates that thoughts have very physical energies and effects. It also demonstrates that thoughts and emotions affect your personal energy level—and your health.

We do an experiment in class to demonstrate just how toxic negative emotions can be. Students scan the solar plexus chakra of an angry person and then scan a piece of pork. (Later in this chapter, you'll read that pork is extremely dirty energetically, and you're advised to eliminate it from your diet.) The solar plexus of the angry person always feels much dirtier, heavier, and stickier than the pork.

Cutting Cords

You establish energetic cords automatically with whatever you turn your attention to. These cords are particularly tenacious when your subject of attention evokes a strong emotion, either positive or negative. Cords attach you to your spouse, family, job, friends, etc. Bundles of these cords extend outward from your energy aura. They can connect to any point in your energy aura, but they frequently attach at the front and back solar plexus chakras because these chakras control the emotions. Cords connecting you to a person or situation that evokes a strong negative emotion, such as worry, fear, anxiety, or anger, lead to energetic contamination, so it is advisable to cut *all* cords periodically, at least once in the evening. It takes only seconds, but it produces a quick sense of relief and lightness. One Pranic Healing practitioner, Arnon Davidovici, uses cord-cutting to regain mental clarity after a long day. Says Arnon: "As the stresses of the day begin to wear on me and I notice that my actions and decisions become less objective and clear, I cut any cords that I don't want connected to me. Immediately, I feel like a different person. I know who I am and what I need to be doing. I make my decisions with more ease and clarity, and I interact with people without external influences and stresses." Many healers use cord-cutting to remove the attachment they make to their patients. Jason J. Wilson, a Minneapolis chiropractor, notes that cord-cutting is "extremely relieving" for him. It gives him more energy, since he is no longer contaminated by the backflow of dirty energy through cords left intact with his patients.

Cord-Cutting to Help Children

"I've found cord-cutting to be particularly helpful in relieving anxiety in children. Our older daughter didn't want to go to kindergarten on her first day. She was still 'attached' to her mother. But after my wife cut the cord between Genevie and her mom, Genevie marched right off to school without any more tears."

—*Master Stephen Co*

EXERCISE 10–B: *Cutting Cords*

Stand for this exercise. No warm-up is necessary, but you should invoke, take a couple of pranic breaths, shake your hands a few times, and silently establish your intent to cut these cords.

1. Put your hands in the slightly cupped general sweeping position. Place one hand above and slightly in front of your head and place the other hand down at your side but curving slightly inward toward your body (Figure 10–1). It will be as if you were holding a large ball in front of you. Most people put their dominant or energizing hand at the top.
2. Imagine beams of light projecting from your fingertips long enough to sweep across the front of your body.
3. Now sweep down with your top hand while sweeping up from below with your other hand. You can dip your knees in order to sweep across your legs in front. Imagine that you are gathering together all these cords, from the bottom of your feet to the top of your head, that are connected to various parts of your energy aura.
4. Pull them together into one bundle in front of your front solar plexus chakra. You should be able to feel them as your hands get about 8 to 12 inches apart. Then grasp the cords in the hand that swept up from below (Figure 10–2).

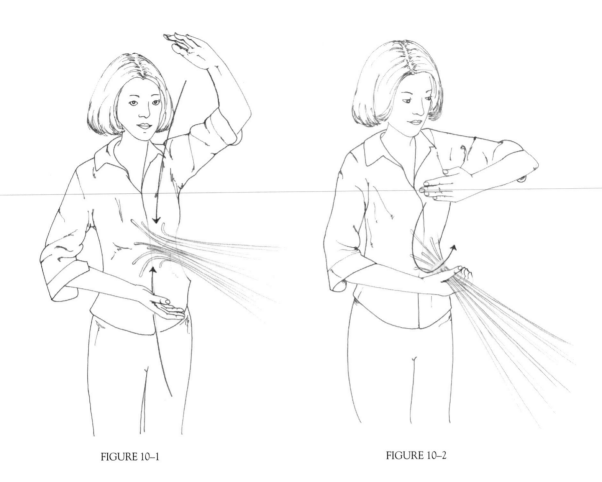

FIGURE 10–1   FIGURE 10–2

5. Cut through the cords forcefully with a brisk karate chop motion with your dominant or top hand. You may wish to visualize the edge of your hand as a sharp serrated knife. Make three cuts close to your body at the front solar plexus. Then clear the cords away, throwing them off to the side. If you have salt water handy, throw them into salt water. If not, just use the green-flame-in-a-bucket visualization.

6. Visualize a picture of your back. Make it one-third real-life size for ease.

7. Place one hand above your visualized head and one hand below your visualized feet.

8. Sweep and gather the cords into a bundle at your back solar plexus chakra in the same manner, then cut them with three sharp motions. Throw them into the same bundle.

9. Now be aware of your crown, and project violet or electric violet prana for about five seconds into the bundle of cords to neutralize them.

Closing and Strengthening Your Aura

This technique, from an advanced Pranic Healing practice called *psychic self-defense*, enables you to close and strengthen your energy aura to make it less susceptible to contamination by the negative words or emotions of others. Like pranic breathing, closing your aura is extremely simple, but very powerful. Pranic Healing student Naila Vavra uses it regularly. "I deal with many people daily, and closing the aura has proven to be very effective at shielding me from people's negativity," she says. "Recently, someone approached me using offensive language. I quickly closed my aura and stood slightly sideways to the person. In less than a minute, the person just walked off, mumbling to himself." You may want to perform it just before or even during a meeting with someone who you know often expresses himself in a negative or angry way. Two variations of this powerful exercise follow.

EXERCISE 10–C: *Closing and Strengthening Your Aura*

Both variations can be performed while standing or sitting.

Variation 1

1. Put your tongue on your palate.
2. Invoke.
3. Form an intent to close your aura to all negative thoughts, emotions, and words.
4. Cross your arms. (This closes the upper half of your aura.)
5. Cross your legs. (This closes the lower half of your aura.)

This posture automatically closes your aura to negativity. It also makes you more naturally resistant to people trying to influence you. This posture is universally interpreted as defensive, however, so you may want to try this subtler, but just as effective, variation:

Variation 2

1. Put your tongue on your palate.
2. Invoke.
3. Tap your *ajna* chakra (center of will) and mentally affirm with full conviction, "Aura! You will shrink and compact *now!*" Repeat three times.
4. After the danger or conflict has passed, say, "Aura, normalize." (This prevents any negative thoughts and emotions from being trapped in a tightly compacted aura.)

Both cord-cutting and closing/strengthening your aura make you much less susceptible to energetic contamination from other people. Practice them regularly.

PROPER DIET

To apply energetic hygiene to your diet, strive to eat food that is physically and energetically clean. Physically, your food should be as free as possible of dirt, germs, and toxins. Energetically, it should be "clean" and "light" when you scan and feel it; it should not feel "sticky" and "heavy."

Table 10–I contains a food hierarchy that classifies food categories from the energetically cleanest to dirtiest.

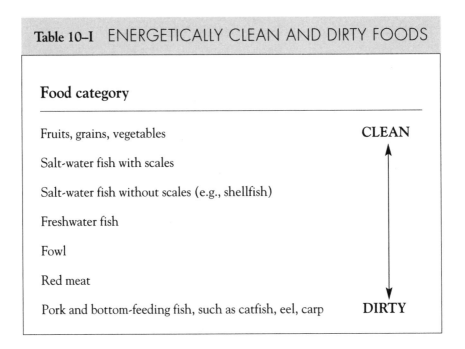

Table 10–I ENERGETICALLY CLEAN AND DIRTY FOODS

Food category

Fruits, grains, vegetables	**CLEAN**
Salt-water fish with scales	↑
Salt-water fish without scales (e.g., shellfish)	
Freshwater fish	
Fowl	
Red meat	↓
Pork and bottom-feeding fish, such as catfish, eel, carp	**DIRTY**

Fruits, grains, and vegetables are energetically clean because they are close to the ultimate sources of prana: the sun, air, and earth. They have more prana, and their prana is more refined, which means you can absorb it more easily.

Meat is farther away from the ultimate sources of prana because animals have to eat plants or other animals; they get their energy indirectly. As a result, the prana in meat is more gross. The particles of energy are dirtier, larger, and less refined, which means your body has to work harder to extract energy from meat. The prana in meat is also gross because the fear and trauma experienced by an animal when it is being slaughtered is trapped in its body. When you consume that meat, those negative emotional energies are absorbed by your solar plexus chakras and your aura. Additionally, meat is often physically dirty due to the heavy addition of growth hormones to livestock feed and drugs given to animals to prevent illness and disease. A person with a meat-heavy diet tends to have a generally dirty aura. It may be large when you scan it, particularly the basic and navel chakras, but it's congested.

Certain sects of ancient *chi kung* masters and martial artists purposefully supplemented their training and energy-development exercises with a diet that was very heavy in meat in order to develop their basic chakras and build up physical power for combat. They were indeed very energized and very powerful physically. In fact, they needed very little sleep. But because their energy bodies were filled with gross, unrefined energy, they were also very unbalanced energetically and emotionally. Their energy bodies had little room to absorb any higher-quality, refined spiritual prana. They also tended to die at a relatively young age, because their bodies were just worn out by the high level of contamination and gross energy.

Recommendations for an Energetically Clean Diet

Here are some dietary recommendations made solely on the basis of maximizing your energy and health. They have no connection or relevance to any particular religions or other beliefs. Adopt them as you feel comfortable.

- Increase your consumption of clean foods that are high in energy, particularly fruits, grains, and vegetables.
- Cut back or minimize energetically dirty foods.
- Eliminate pork, catfish, and eel; they are energetically very dirty foods.
- Choose fresh, natural, or organic foods over preserved or processed foods; they contain more prana.
- Don't overcook your food; excessive heat neutralizes prana.
- Minimize your consumption of microwaved foods. While microwaving may not affect the nutritional value of food, it does reduce significantly its energetic potency.
- Consume alcohol in moderation. Wine or beer in small amounts has a cleansing effect on food due to its slight alcohol content. Hard liquor drains away prana; there's too much alcohol in it.

EXERCISE 10–D: *Scanning Food for Cleanliness and Energy*

(*Note:* This is a slightly more advanced technique. We recommend that you attempt it only after you become a proficient scanner.)

Before you begin, obtain the following: a fresh piece of regular fruit, a fresh piece of organic fruit, a slice of whole wheat bread, a piece of unfrozen fish, a piece of red meat, and a piece of pork. Perform your standard warm-up.

1. Silently form your intent to scan and compare the cleanliness and energetic potencies of these foods.

2. Put the piece of regular fruit on the table. Keep the others away from the table. Scan the fruit from several angles, and note the depth and strength of its energy aura. After you scan a few times, slowly sweep away some of the energy into your scanning hand, and feel it in your hand. Roll it between your fingers. You may have a sensation like a light vibration or a feeling of lightness. Shake your scanning hand downward a few times before moving on to scan the next food.

3. Scan the piece of organic fruit, noting the depth and strength of its energy. Then sweep away and feel some of its energy. The light vibration should be stronger. Shake your scanning hand a few times.

4. Perform the same routine on the piece of bread. Depending on the brand and its freshness, it should have a feeling close to that of the original piece of fruit. Shake your hand after each piece of food.

5. Scan the fish, the red meat, and the pork. The energy of each will feel progressively heavier and denser, maybe sticky.

6. Spray your hands with alcohol.

7. Now pick one or two items that felt particularly clean and strong to you and put them in the microwave for about 45 seconds. Take them out and scan them. You will feel a substantial drop in energy.

You may wish to try scanning different types of food and different brands, and scanning food before and after it is prepared by different methods.

Cleaning Your Food

Since no food, not even organic produce, is completely free of contamination, it is a good idea to clean and energize your food before you eat it. Two routines are presented here: one for use before eating and one for use "retroactively," for those times when you can't discreetly clean your food. Nearly everyone who practices food cleaning finds that their food actually tastes different and better: light, clean, and more flavorful, instead of thick and heavy.

Have your container of salt water and your alcohol sprayer handy.

EXERCISE 10–E: *Energetically Cleaning Your Food*

Perform your standard warm-up.

1. Put your awareness on your throat chakra for a second, then energize your food with light green for 10 seconds. Shake your energizing hand for a few seconds.
2. Put your awareness on your crown chakra again for a second, then energize your food with light violet for 10 seconds. The quick green-then-violet sequence loosens dirty energy. Shake your energizing hand for a few seconds again.
3. Sweep the food with white prana about 10 times or until it feels clean. Throw the dirty energy into salt water, if you have it handy, or into a visualization of a green flame in a bucket.
4. Put your awareness on your crown, and energize the food with violet for about 10 seconds.
5. If you have time, energize also with electric violet. Allow the energy to penetrate into the food for 1 to 2 minutes before eating.
6. Rescan your food. Its energy will be cleaner, stronger, and lighter.

EXERCISE 10–F: *"Retroactive" Food Cleansing*

You can use this technique if you have to eat energetically dirty food and are unable to perform the cleansing routine above. (Perhaps you're at a dinner party where they're serving red meat or pork, and you don't wish to offend your host.) You should perform this technique as soon as you are able after eating.

This technique uses Colon Cleanse, a psyllium product that helps flush toxins from the digestive system. See "For Further Reference" section for information on where to get it.

Perform your standard warm-up.

1. Take a glassful of Colon Cleanse, as per the directions on the label.
2. Perform local sweeping on the stomach and abdomen with green and violet alternately (two sets of five with green, spray hands, then two sets of five violet, until you reach 40 sweeps total).
3. Perform local sweeping on the front solar plexus chakra with green and violet alternately (40 sweeps total).

4. Perform local sweeping on the back solar plexus chakra with green and violet alternately (40 sweeps total). Option: Since dirty food can contaminate your entire energy body, you may wish to precede steps 5 through 9 with a quick general sweeping routine. The technique will be quite effective even without general sweeping, though.

5. Perform local sweeping on the navel chakra with green and violet alternately (40 sweeps total).

6. Perform local sweeping on the liver with green and violet alternately (40 sweeps total).

7. Energize the navel chakra with white prana for ten cycles of pranic breathing.

Cleaning and Energizing Your Drinking Water

Although bottled and filtered waters are better than tap water, even purified water contains some energetic contamination. Clean your drinking water if you have time. You can also charge it up with prana to make it even more healthful.

EXERCISE 10–G: *Cleaning and Energizing Your Drinking Water*

Pour your drinking water into a large glass jar or bottle. Plastic containers are made from petrochemical byproducts and are energetically dirty. Mountain spring water and filtered water are preferable to tap water; however, the steps below clean and energize even tap water.

Perform your standard warm-up.

1. Before sweeping and cleaning, scan the water and note the size and strength of its energetic field.

2. Sweep the water with light violet for 20 cycles and dispose of any contamination in a pan of salt water, or use the visualized green-flame-in-a-bucket technique.

3. Energize the water with light violet for four pranic breathing cycles while forming a strong intent that the water be highly energized. Stabilize and lock in the energy by energizing it with light blue. Stabilize again.

4. Leave the bottle or jar out in sun for one to two days to absorb solar prana.

5. Rescan in a couple of days. You should see a substantial difference in the size and strength of its energetic field.

Short-cut: If you don't have time, you can either clean and energize the water, or leave the jar in the sun for two days. Then stabilize.

Herbs and Supplements

Certain herbs and food supplements produce dramatic cleansing and energizing effects because they contain large amounts of concentrated colored prana. Table 10–II includes some of these tested supplements, along with recommended brands and dosages. (*Note:* Anyone with cancer, AIDS, or any serious autoimmune disorder should *not* take cleansing or energizing herbs or supplements without their doctor's approval. Some accelerate the diseases.)

EXERCISE 10–H: *Comparing the Potency of Vitamins, Herbs and Supplements*

You can use the food scanning technique (Exercise 10–D) to measure the relative cleanliness and energetic potency of vitamins, herbs, and supplements.

Perform your standard warm-up.

1. Silently form your intent to scan and compare the cleanliness and energetic potencies of these vitamins, herbs, and supplements.
2. Scan the containers or bottles one at a time, and compare the feeling. The product with the strongest energy aura (and without any feeling of heaviness or stickiness) is the strongest and cleanest for you.

As you refine your scanning ability and focus your intent, you can do this technique discreetly even in the grocery store.

Scanning to Determine Energetic Potency of Food and Food Supplements

"Grandmaster Choa Kok Sui always scans the products on the shelf before he buys them. One day while I was in a health food store with him, he asked me to scan a bottle of barley grass tablets and a bottle of wheat grass tablets and tell him which had more energy. I scanned and picked out the barley grass bottle because its aura was twice as big and felt dense and tightly packed. He commended me for the proper choice."

—*Master Stephen Co*

Table 10-II	ENERGIZING AND CLEANSING HERBS AND SUPPLEMENTS

Herb or Supplement	Effect	Prana It Contains	How to Take It	Preferred Process or Brand
Blue-green algae	Cleansing	Multicolored; primarily green	Pills or powder	Klamath
"Green foods" like wheat grass and barley grass	Strong cleansing and energizing	Multicolored; primarily green	Pills or powder	Cold- or dry-pressed; Green Magma
Garlic	Strong cleansing	Orange	Capsules, gel caps; 3,000 mg/day	Any brand of pure garlic; deodorized is fine
Ginseng	Energizing; increases chakra size, expands aura	Multicolored; mostly reddish; high-quality has gold prana	Pills or liquid; ½ g per day, twice daily	Korean Red or Chinese Red
Royal jelly	Energizing	Red, yellow	As per instructions on container	The fresher the better; no recommended brand
Bee propolis	Cleansing	Green, blue	As per instructions on container	The fresher the better; no recommended brand
Bee pollen	Energizing	Multicolored	1–2 g per day	The fresher the better; no recommended brand
Psyllium products	Cleansing stomach, intestines, front and back solar plexus, and navel chakras	Green, orange	As per instructions on bottle	Colon Cleanse or similar product with pure psyllium husks; no sugar, starches, additives

PHYSICAL EXERCISE

Vigorous physical exercise cleans the body's energy channels. Running, aerobics, weight-lifting, tennis, or any activity that gets your joints and blood moving also gets your energy moving. Physical exertion tones you not only physically but energetically because it dislodges and expels energetic congestion. Tai chi and the martial arts, in particular, are excellent for energetic hygiene, but any exercise will cleanse your energy body.

Below is a set of mild stretches and exercises developed specifically to cleanse your energy body. They can be used as a warm-up to a more vigorous exercise program, if you practice one, or alone as part of your energy work and self-healing. They're particularly good for those who are physically restricted or don't have the time to exercise, because they give you maximum energy benefit in minimum time and with little exertion. These exercises can also serve as your pre- and post-meditation exercise routine. Used before meditation, they open up your energy channels to prepare them to get the prana flowing through them. Used after meditation, they prevent energy congestion. Don't be misled by their simplicity. They're powerful.

The entire routine takes about 10 minutes.

(*Note*: Don't strain. Your movements should be smooth and gentle. Don't stretch any joint beyond your comfortable range of motion. The exercises outline the maximum normal stretch. If you are physically restricted or have pain in a particular area, don't stretch beyond the point of comfort. As always, check with your physician or health care practitioner before beginning any exercise program.)

Perform these exercises standing up in loose clothing and with a relaxed posture.

EXERCISE 10–1: *Cleansing Physical Exercises*

1. Eye rotations: Roll your eyes 12 times clockwise, then 12 times counterclockwise. (Your orientation is as if a clock were on your body with its face outward.)
2. Neck rotations: Beginning with your face forward, gently twist your head left and then right 12 times. At its farthest point on each turn, your chin should be roughly over your collar bone. Then gently move your head up and down 12 times. At its farthest point downward, your chin should be near your chest. At its farthest point backward, your head should be as far back as you can comfortably go.
3. Shoulder rotations: With your arms fully outstretched to the side, rotate your arms forward 12 times, pivoting at the shoulder. Then rotate them backward 12 times.

4. Wrist rotations: With your arms fully stretched forward, roll your wrists 12 times to the outside, then 12 times to the inside.

5. Hand looseners: With your arms fully stretched forward, open and close your hands 12 times.

6. Torso twists: With your feet planted and your arms outstretched and parallel to the ground, twist your trunk 12 times to the right and to the left. Twist as far as you can comfortably without straining. As you twist, gradually bring your arms down so that by your 12th twist they're about at waist level.

7. Hip rotations: With your hands on your hips and your knees slightly bent, rotate your hips 12 times in a clockwise circle, then 12 times counterclockwise. (Clockwise is as if a clock were lying on the ground at your feet with its face upward.) The hip rotation is also called the "brain exercise" because it stimulates energy from the lower chakras and drives it upward to the brain.

8. Quarter-squats: Bending slightly at the knees, do 100 quarter-squats. A full squat means your buttocks are almost resting on your heels as you come down. A quarter-squat means you're *slightly* dipping your knees. The quarter-squat highly activates your basic chakra, which gives you more energy.

9. Knee rotations: Put your legs together and bend slightly at the knees. Place your hands on your kneecaps and rotate your legs (Figure 10–3). Rotate them 12 times clockwise and 12 times counterclockwise.

10. Ankle rotations: Standing on your right leg, lift up your left leg and extend it slightly. Rotate your ankle 12 times to the left and 12 times to the right. Then perform the exercise with your right ankle.

11. Shake in place: Now simply bounce on the balls of your feet and shake your arms and hands for about 30 seconds.

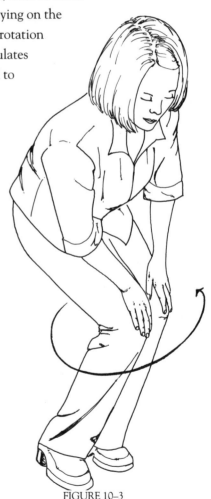

FIGURE 10–3

CLEAN HOME AND WORK ENVIRONMENT

Certain places are intrinsically dirtier than others. The room of a sick person, a typical hospital, an office with poor circulation and fluorescent lights, and a building in which the occupants are smokers are all energetically dirty environments. If you spend time in these surroundings, you are exposed to greater-than-average energetic contamination. Thus, you may need to practice energetic hygiene more diligently and more regularly—for example, cutting cords and performing general self-sweeping. You can also directly clean the area.

Use standard preparation steps before any of these techniques.

EXERCISE 10–J: *Cleaning a Room or Building of Dirty Energy*

1. *Burn incense.* Burn a stick or cone of incense in the rooms of your house or work area. Sandalwood is the most cleansing incense; it contains much high-quality green prana. If you prefer different fragrances, however, lavender incense contains blue-violet prana, and sage incense contains green, blue, and violet prana.
2. *Chant "OM" or "amen."* Chant the mantra "OM" or "amen" in the room for 20 minutes. Both mantras disperse dirty energy, which is why they're universally used as part of many meditation routines to clear the mind of thoughts. You'll learn more about OM in the next chapter on meditation. As an alternative, you can play the Grandmaster Choa Kok Sui OM CD. (For more information see "Pranic Healing Classes" section.)
3. *Open all windows and curtains to let fresh air and sunlight in.* An easy way to clean a house or room energetically is to open the windows and curtains allowing cleansing solar and air prana to flood inside. An hour or two a day should be sufficient for moderate residual contamination.
4. *Spray the area with salt water from a sprayer.* Mix a few tablespoons of salt with a cup of water in a sprayer with a fine misting capability. Shake to dissolve the salt. Walk through a room spraying the salt and water into the air, allowing the droplets to filter down to the floor. Just as salt water breaks down the dirty energy that you sweep from your own aura, it also effectively cleans a room or building.
5. *Loud clapping.* Loud, purposeful clapping with intent can break up and disperse dirty energy in a room. Go into a room, form a clear intent to dispel the dirty energy, and walk through the area clapping 10 to 30 times, depending on the size of the room. One clap per second is a good pace.

It may be difficult to perform some of these routines in your work area, so here is a technique that can be employed for either home or work:

6. *Sweep the room or area with electric violet.* Perform your standard warm-up. You will need a bowl of salt water, or you can use the green flame technique. You'll also need your alcohol sprayer.

    • Visualize your house or workplace very small, about a foot in total area, in front of you. Make the visualization as clear as you can.

    • Form an intent to scan the house or area to determine if there is any dirty energy, and then scan it. Be aware of any sensations of stickiness or heaviness, just as you did when you scanned your own body.

    • Imagine electric violet beams projecting from the fingertips of your scanning hand, and sweep the house or area with the beams. After five passes, throw the dirty energy into the bowl of salt water.

    • Perform 10 total sets of five sweeps of the area. Spray your scanning hand with alcohol after every 10 passes. You can also spray the visualization a few times with alcohol.

    • Rescan the house. It should be much cleaner than it was before you started.

SALT

One of the most effective energetic hygiene steps is also one of the simplest, most inexpensive, and least esoteric: taking advantage of the natural cleansing ability of salt. Since it is filled with green prana, salt quickly breaks down dirty energy. You've already learned one application of salt: flicking your hands into a bowl of salt water as you sweep. Here are some others.

EXERCISE 10–K: *A Cleansing Salt Bath*

For this exercise, you'll need a 26-ounce container of table salt. It doesn't make any difference energetically if the salt has iodine in it ("iodized") or not ("plain"). But it should be regular salt and not Epsom salts, which do not have the same cleansing ability.

1. Draw a tub full of warm water and pour the entire container of salt into the water. Soak in the bath for 15 to 20 minutes. Sink down into the water so that your body is com-

pletely submerged up to your chin. If you sit up in the tub and read while taking this bath, your upper body chakras will not be cleansed.

2. After you are finished, take a regular shower with soap and shampoo.

You will emerge feeling calm, light, and refreshed. You may also experience heightened sexual desire afterward. A salt bath thoroughly cleanses the sex and basic chakras, which frequently get contaminated during the day, particularly if your job involves a lot of sitting.

How frequently you take a salt bath depends on how contaminated you get. If you work in a stressful, energetically dirty environment (indoors, with little fresh air and light, and under fluorescent lights) or with sick or contaminated people (in a hospital), you may need to take a salt bath more frequently than others. In general, though, twice a week is sufficient.

If you wish to make your bath even more cleansing, add up to 10 drops of lavender oil. Lavender contains blue-violet prana, and when added to a salt bath, makes for an even more effective and pleasantly fragrant bath. For a variation that has even greater cleansing ability as well as a different fragrance, add up to 10 drops of tea tree oil or eucalyptus oil to your salt bath. Tea tree oil has green and eucalyptus orange prana; both have a powerful cleansing effect.

(*Note:* Do not combine two of these three oils and especially do not combine all three. Mixing them will pull out too much energy, even clean energy.)

EXERCISE 10–L: *Salt Shower Instead of a Salt Bath*

If you don't have access to a bathtub, you can still cleanse yourself with salt. Simply take a container of fine salt with you into the shower, pour a small portion into your palm and then rub it onto your skin, one body part at a time. Pay special attention to your front and back solar plexus chakras. Rub the salt on in counterclockwise circles. Allow it to stay on the skin for about 15 seconds, then wash it off. A salt shower is not as effective as a salt bath, but it certainly will cleanse away the portions of heavy energetic contamination.

EXERCISE 10–M: *Making and Using "Salt Soap"*

Salt soap can be used in the shower or to wash off your hands after a self-healing or energy practice session.

To make salt soap, all you need is a container of salt and a bottle of liquid soap. Any brand will do. Many people like antibacterial soaps, but others feel they wash away beneficial as well as harmful bacteria.

1. Pour out one-third of the liquid soap. (You can save it in another bottle and add it back to the first bottle as you use it up.) Add enough salt to the bottle that the resulting mixture is slightly gritty but not so thick that it won't pump out of the bottle if you're using a bottle that has a pump on it. To make it even more powerful, add 20 drops of pure lavender essential oil.

2. Shake before using, and you've got a powerful energetic cleansing potion that you can use any time.

A Cleansing Swim

This isn't really an exercise; it's more a tip on how to take advantage of the biggest natural salt bath available, the ocean. Even though shorelines are polluted to varying degrees, the amount of salt in sea water gives you a tremendous opportunity to clean away dirty energy. If you have access to the sea, take advantage of it. It really works. One Pranic Healing student tells the story of how, before her involvement with Pranic Healing, she contracted a serious blood infection following gastrointestinal surgery. After her discharge from the hospital, she was given heavy doses of antibiotics and told to stay in bed for a month. As she contemplated her situation, she recalled a story her husband had told her. He had a cut that had turned gangrenous, so his grandmother took him to the ocean and instructed him to stay in the water all day. He did, and the following day, the gangrene was gone. So, the instructor decided to try the same approach. She booked a flight to Mexico and sat in the ocean for much of the next ten days. Her infection was completely healed.

ENERGETIC HYGIENE CHECKLIST

Presented below are recommendations for incorporating energetic hygiene into your life. As you practice this routine regularly, you will experience a cleaner and stronger flow of prana through your energy body.

Emotional Regulation

1. Self-awareness and higher-level thinking, as needed.
2. General self-sweeping two to three times per week, using the variation that's most effective for you.

3. Daily practice of pranic breathing.
4. Cut cords nightly, or as needed through the day.
5. Close and strengthen your aura, as you are confronted by negative people or as needed.
6. Do the general stress-relief technique (Exercise 9–F) twice weekly or as needed.

Diet

1. Avoid pork, eel, and catfish; minimize red meat.
2. Increase your consumption of clean foods that are high in energy, particularly fruits, grains, and vegetables.
3. Minimize your consumption of microwaved foods.
4. Consume alcohol in moderation (no hard liquor; no more than a glass or two of wine or beer per day).
5. Clean and energize your food and drinking water (Exercises 10–E and 10–G) whenever possible.
6. Add herbs and supplements to your diet as necessary. (Consider taking Colon Cleanse to help keep solar plexus chakras clean.)

Physical Exercise

1. Perform the Cleansing Physical Exercise (Exercise 10–I) at least once daily in the morning.
2. Do any type of physical exercise routine that you like or that your physician suggests.
3. Do any tai chi, yoga, or martial art that you like or are physically able to do.

Clean Home and Work Environment

Clean your home and work area (Exercise 10–J) twice weekly, or as needed throughout the week, with your preferred method.

Salt

Take a salt bath (Exercise 10–K) two to three times a week, or as needed, according to your level of contamination.

SIX STEPS DAILY PRACTICE ROUTINE—UPDATE

You may, at this point in your development, wish to combine all your exercises into one long morning or evening routine. Here is one possible sequence:

1. Invoke for guidance and protection.
2. Cut cords.
3. Cleansing physical exercises.
4. Pranic breathing.
5. Direct clearing techniques, as needed.
6. Standard warm-up.
7. Hand sensitivity, scanning, sweeping, energizing practice.
8. Special exercises: general self-sweeping, general stress reduction, work/house cleaning, etc.

Add the other elements of energetic hygiene to your daily routine as you are able, or as you see fit.

In the next chapter you'll learn the fifth of the six steps to self-healing, *meditation*, to help relax your mind and energize your body.

CHAPTER 11

Easy Ways to Put Your Mind at Ease— Meditations for Peace and Stillness

"My introduction to meditation was with Grandmaster Choa's Meditation on Twin Hearts. When I was guided in this meditation for the first time, I was amazed at the experience I had. I knew that meditation was supposed to induce a sense of peace and tranquility in one's thoughts and emotions, but with this meditation I experienced so much more!

"At the beginning of the meditation, when you are guided in thinking of a happy event, I could immediately feel a warm loving feeling emanating from my heart and overwhelming me with joy. This joy then seemed to travel throughout my body. I could feel waves of energy moving through me and relaxing me so much that all the different thoughts running through my head began to disappear.

"As the meditation continued and I focused on my heart and crown chakras, I could instantly feel a tingling sensation moving through the center of my chest and into my head. I could only describe the experience as 'liquid light' moving up into my head, out of my crown, and then pouring back down over me with more energy, as if I were under a huge waterfall of light! It moved through my body and removed all the stress and frustrations I had been feeling through the day. I was feeling light and clean!

"When we blessed the earth through our hands, everything I was feeling was intensified, and I felt tremendous bliss! Compassion and love overwhelmed me. I could feel energy pouring into me through my crown, and my hands began to feel warm; they throbbed with energy. The meditation left me with a feeling of happiness that lasted for days!

"The Meditation on Twin Hearts always leaves me with a great feeling of unconditional

love, peace, clarity, lovingkindness, and wholeness. Negative people and stressful situations don't affect me as easily as they used to, and my ability to remain centered, at peace, and objective has dramatically increased! The Meditation on Twin Hearts is a powerful tool in helping ourselves to live a happier, healthier, more positive life!"

—Karla M. Alvarez, Chino, California

Here is the most difficult exercise in the entire book.

Put yourself into a comfortable position, either sitting or lying down. Close your eyes and relax your body. Use the sequential relaxation from the self-awareness exercise (Exercise 3–A) if you wish. Perform six cycles of pranic breathing to help relax further.

Now let your mind go completely blank for one minute. Turn off all your thoughts and sensory impressions. That means no thinking about what you did this morning or what you'll do tonight, no hearing favorite songs running through your head, no seeing images of loved ones, no feeling what's going on in your body as you do in self-awareness. Keep your mind blank and your thoughts perfectly still for 60 seconds.

Most people find it difficult to keep this state of blankness and stillness for 10 seconds, let alone a full minute. Many are simply unable at all to turn off the pictures, sounds, and impressions that flow through their "monkey mind," the name that ancient Oriental spiritual masters gave our unconscious because it flits from thought to thought the way a jittery monkey darts from tree branch to tree branch. This mental chatter diverts our attention, consumes energy, and creates tension in both our mind and body.

You can learn to control that stream of chatter through the fifth of the six steps to self-healing, *meditation*, which brings about mental and physical relaxation as well as a host of healthful, energetic benefits. Meditation is a blend of concentration and sensitivity. Concentration is will, the ability to have prolonged focus or single-point concentration. Sensitivity is attentiveness, the ability to have prolonged awareness, or quiet, watchful sensing. Thus, meditation trains the mind to engage in a sustained mental concentration on a single point while remaining open to impressions that come from within.

THE BENEFITS OF MEDITATION

The benefits of meditation range from the simple and obvious (greater physical relaxation) to the subtle and less known (inner stillness), but they all support your greater goals—increased energy and improved health. Here are the principal benefits of meditation.

1. *Mental and Physical Relaxation.* At its most basic, meditation is a mental exercise that helps you achieve deep relaxation of mind and body. It begins with deep breathing and purposeful physical relaxation, one body part at a time. This progressive relaxation leads to slower, deeper breathing, which in turn promotes further mental and physical relaxation. Finally, as your mind becomes even more relaxed, the chatter of your monkey mind subsides, which leads to a deep healing state.

   Meditation helps you circumvent the "fight-or-flight" response, a set of involuntary bodily reactions that include increased adrenaline production, heart rate, and blood pressure. Originating from the same "old" part of the brain as the unconscious mind's survival instinct, these physiological reactions developed to prepare our prehistoric ancestors to "fight" a threat to their existence or to take "flight" and run away from it. Psychological researchers have discovered that stress and other negative emotions, such as fear, anger, and anxiety, produce the same physiological, neurological, and endocrinological changes in your body that the fight-or-flight response does. Furthermore, when you endure stress for a long period, or when you live in a constant state of fear, anger, or anxiety, you experience a sustained fight-or-flight reaction, which is not good for you. The fight-or-flight response was hardwired into our brain for short-term use only. Frequent or extended adrenaline surges and increased heart rate and blood pressure can lead to serious health problems. Biofeedback studies have demonstrated that meditation produces physiological changes that are the *opposite* of the fight-or-flight reaction, including reduced heart rate and blood pressure and regulated production of adrenaline. These physiological changes are also associated with mental and physical relaxation.

2. *Sharpened Mental Acuity.* Since meditation involves prolonged attention of the mind on a particular point, most people find that it sharpens their mental faculties in general and even enables them to sustain their attention when performing everyday tasks. After meditating for a while, for instance, you may find you can read for longer periods while retaining more of what you read. Or you may find you have an increased facility with numbers. It's not that meditation makes you smarter or more intelligent. It's just that you'll be more relaxed, patient, and able to use more of your mind.

3. *Objectivity.* Regular meditation gives you perspective on yourself, your habits, and your behaviors. You come to see yourself from the outside; you acquire objectivity and conscious-unconscious dissociation. This detachment from your thoughts, impressions, and emotions diminishes their power over you and increases your power over them. You starve them of attention and energy and gain a firm sense of control over your unconscious mind.

   Zen Buddhism views the mind as a turbulent pool of water. If you swish your hand in a pool, for example, you stir up the mud at the bottom and make it more difficult to see. But if you sit quietly and observe, the mud will settle; you can see clearly. Similarly, if you act aggressively and try to use your willpower to change unwanted thoughts, reactions, and behaviors or suppress negative emotions and thoughts, all you do is "muddy the pool" of your mind. You can't change an unconscious thought or clear a negative emotion with a conscious, forceful effort. Your unconscious mind will fight you, clamp down further on those negative emotions, or bury limiting beliefs even deeper in your body.

Optimal insight and change are best achieved through calm objectivity.

4. *Mindfulness.* As you meditate, you learn to keep your attention on each discrete moment as it presents itself to you. You note each breath, thought, and external impression that registers upon your senses objectively and without judgment. You notice and let go of frustration or anger. You gently bring your attention back to your breathing or some other point of focus and remain aware. This is the essence of mindfulness: moment-to-moment awareness that allows you to have true reflection, not only on the inner workings of your thoughts, but also your daily existence.

Most of us lead lives that are too hurried and filled with nonessential chores. We have lengthy personal to-do lists that we make without full consideration of their true value to us. Our lives have inadequate reflection, high stress, little peace, and frequently numerous mental and physical ailments. When you incorporate mindfulness into meditation and daily life, however, you see how many of these activities are actually mind*less* and unimportant. Mindfulness enables you to see and choose meaningful actions and activities and then to appreciate better the actions and activities you do choose. By making time for meditation, you make more time for real life in your daily life.

5. *Stillness.* Stillness is an inner state brought about by becoming aware of the space between your thoughts and focusing on this gap between your impressions. Just as retention, the pause between inhalation and exhalation, is the secret to a powerful pranic breath, the stillness or gap between thoughts is the key to meditation's physical, mental, and energetic health benefits.

As you progress in meditation, your goal is to stretch out that gap, that stillness, and then maintain your awareness of it. The reason is simple: When there is chaos in the mind—through constant chatter and the presence of negative emotions, fears, and anxieties—true mental and physical health is not possible. Nor are higher goals such as self-realization. But stillness makes these goals attainable.

Zen masters used to pose this query to their students: Which is more important, the vase or the space the vase surrounds into which we place the flowers? The answer is that both are equally important. You can't pour water or place flowers into a solid object.

And space needs form around it to be useful. In the same way that aspiring Zen priests were taught to appreciate the space between solid objects, meditation teaches you to be aware of the silence, the stillness, between thoughts.

6. *More Overall Energy and Improved Health.* Meditation helps free you from the negative emotions and limiting beliefs that are the root of many physical ailments. The ability to maintain a state of stillness, even for a brief period of time, produces powerful energetic and health changes. The most notable of these occurs when, during Meditation on Twin Hearts, prolonged stillness enables you to draw in through your crown chakra a great quantity of prana. This is healing prana of the highest quality.

Here is how one relatively new Pranic Healing student, Valarie Anderson, explained the difference these meditations have made in her life:

I can't imagine life without Pranic Healing and the meditations that are taught along with it. Two years ago I made the decision to end my marriage. Although I know my choice was the best thing I could do for myself and my child, the process of divorce, reestablishing a new life and home, and bearing the emotional and financial burden alone was terrifying to me. The amount of psychological stress, emotional pain, and duress I was under at the time was overwhelming. I am a 38-year-old mother with a high-pressure advertising career where I am constantly under deadline. Of course, pending divorce only added to my stress level.

At about this time, I accepted an invitation to a Pranic Healing class. Although I had always steered clear of these kinds of classes, it turned out to be the best invitation I have ever accepted. The lecture on meditation that Master Co gave resonated with familiar truths, practical applications, and intriguing wisdoms. It ended with a Meditation on Twin Hearts that left me embarrassingly teary-eyed but peaceful for the first time in years. I realized that afternoon how dangerously close I was to becoming a bitter, stressed-out, and overly critical and cynical person. That meditation showed me my own true nature, which was the exact opposite of how I was currently existing.

Since then, I have incorporated daily meditations and techniques that are taught by Grandmaster Choa into my daily life. These meditations have given me a clarity and inner wisdom that has given me the peace of mind to deal with the same stresses and responsibilities but from a more empowered place. I now have a bigger picture of my life and place in the world around me and have been wondrously pulled out of the myopic self-centered rat race in which I had been functioning. I even have a better paying and more respectable position within my industry that affords me a schedule to incorporate being a full-time mother to my son. I would have never had the courage, clarity, and strength to make these changes without the focus my meditations give me. The quality of my life has greatly improved because I have a clutter-free mind and the inner strength to create my life daily. It is amazing how much more productive and energetic I am without the mental 'pollutants' I used to carry around in my head. With the meditations I have been practicing, I am a happier individual, and that is reflected in every aspect of my life. The key to our own empowerment truly lies within ourselves, and I am forever grateful to the teachings and meditations that have enabled me to tap into this enrichment and begin living my life to its greatest potential.

GENERAL MEDITATION TIPS

These tips apply both to the Mindfulness Meditation and to the Meditation on Twin Hearts.

1. Meditate at the same time every day, whether in the morning, at lunch, or in the evening. Developing a routine helps your practice produce consistent results.

2. Meditate in the same room or corner of a room. This helps you maintain your routine; it also energizes and sensitizes that room or area, thus making it more conducive to the production of clean prana.

3. Keep your primary meditation area physically and energetically clean. As you meditate more, you become more receptive and sensitive to subtle energy, which means you can more easily become contaminated by an energetically dirty environment. Thus, you should practice good energetic hygiene in your meditation area—for example, by burning incense, playing the OM CD, or using other techniques.

4. Refrain from eating a heavy meal before meditating. Physiologically and energetically, your body is focused on digesting food, which may cause you to get sleepy.

5. Do not meditate out in the sun. The solar prana is too intense.

6. Do not meditate in a state of strong negative emotion, such as anger or fear. Use self-awareness or another clearing technique to diminish the negative emotion before you meditate.

7. Refrain from drinking cold beverages for one hour before and one hour after meditating. Meditation generates prana, which is warm. A cold drink creates a sudden change in the body's temperature and shocks the energy channels.

8. Do not take a shower for 2 hours after meditating. Water washes away the prana you generate during meditation.

9. Perform some type of physical exercise for 5 minutes before and 5 minutes after you

meditate, preferably cleansing physical exercises. As you read in the previous chapter, even mild exercise helps prevent congestion and expel dirty prana from the energy body's meridians and chakras. Feel free to supplement the cleansing physical exercises with a routine of your own preference or design—for instance, a tai chi or *chi kung* set, or even aerobics.

10. Don't fight distractions, noises, or other sensory impressions that may interrupt your meditation. More important, don't allow such disturbances to make you angry. If the dog barks or a car horn honks, note it without reacting, and bring your mind back to the focus of your meditation. Don't give in to the distraction. Don't give it attention and energy. You can blend distractions into your meditation this way:
    - Acknowledge the disturbance objectively and without judgment.
    - Say something to yourself such as "Outside noises and sounds only make my meditation deeper and my concentration more focused."
    - Gently turn your attention back to the focus of your meditation and continue.

MINDFULNESS MEDITATION

In many ways the Mindfulness Meditation is merely a more formalized version of the direct clearing technique of self-awareness (Exercise 3–A). As you perform it, you will recognize the same components: systematic physical relaxation, pranic breathing, letting go, and awareness. A mindfulness meditation simply combines these with single-point concentration for a more focused relaxation effect. One student calls this mindfulness meditation "the most powerful instant remedy for hectic, confused mental or emotional states." Another says it makes him immediately "focused, centered, and quiet."

EXERCISE 11–A: *Mindfulness Meditation*

1. Wear comfortable, loose-fitting clothing, especially around the waist. Take off your shoes. You may want to dim the lights, if you think you can meditate in the dark without falling asleep. You may even want to take the phone off the hook. Eliminate as many outside sensory distractions as you can.
2. Perform one or two sets of the Cleansing Physical Exercises (Exercise 10–I), or perform a light exercise routine of your own choice.
3. Sit in a comfortable chair with your back straight (but not tense) and your feet flat on

the floor. If it's a chair with a back, don't lean back or slouch. (*Note:* If sitting up for 10 to 30 minutes is uncomfortable for you, you can meditate lying down, but lying down may cause you to fall asleep.) Place your hands palms up in your lap. Keep them relaxed.

4. Place your tongue on your palate.

5. Invoke.

6. Close your eyes and perform 10 cycles of pranic breathing. After the initial 10 cycles, let your breathing stay deep throughout the balance of the meditation, but don't be overly concerned about your rhythm. A focus on an internal count can be distracting, but some find that a rhythm or count helps them let go. If you can keep the rhythm, or if you find that using an internal count helps you let go, by all means, use it.

7. Relax your body, one part at a time, as you learned to do in Exercise 3–A. Work in an orderly sequence, either head to toe or toe to head, rather than in a haphazard fashion. This relaxation should take 5 to 10 minutes.

8. Touch the tip of your nose with the forefinger of your dominant (scanning) hand for a count of four, then take it away and place it in your lap.

9. After you take it away, continue your breathing, and keep your awareness lightly on the tip of your nose. Awareness is not willful concentration; it's an open state of sensitivity.

10. After a few minutes touch your navel with the forefinger of your dominant hand, return your hand to your lap, and shift your awareness to your navel. As you do this, you should feel your breath being drawn deeply into the abdomen. Remain aware of the in-and-out movement of your navel as you breathe. (*Note:* If you have high blood pressure, don't focus on your navel; keep your awareness on the tip of your nose. Focusing on the navel also secondarily activates the *meng mein* chakra, which can raise the blood pressure.)

11. After a few moments, shift your awareness to your breathing. Some meditation schools urge students to "watch their breath." This is a directive not so much to visualize the breath moving in and out of the nose in a stream as to be lightly aware of the breath as it enters the nose, travels down into the lungs, and then returns out the nose.

12. Perform a posture check periodically. It's natural for your shoulders to slump a bit. If you find your back rounding or your shoulders slumping, gently assume a more erect posture.

13. Hold your awareness on *one* of the three points—nose, navel, or breathing—throughout the meditation. For beginners, the breath is usually the easiest. Continue with breathing and awareness for 10 minutes. Gradually work up to 30 minutes.

14. When you are finished, slowly move around in your chair a bit. If you feel like you've

been off somewhere or out of your body, bring yourself back. Before you open your eyes, ground yourself. Grounding is the process of rooting yourself energetically to the earth. Together with postmeditation exercises, grounding helps you avoid the "spacey" feeling that often follows meditation. Grounding: While seated, imagine brilliant, white beams of prana emitting from the chakras on the soles of your feel and your basic chakra and beaming 10 feet down into the earth. Hold the intent that this energy flow into the earth for about 30 seconds. As you do this, simply say something like, "I now bless and root myself to Mother Earth."

15. Open your eyes, stretch, and get up and perform your postmeditation exercise routine.

Awareness and Mindfulness in Meditation

"There's a story attributed to the meditation master Eknath Easwaren that nicely illustrates the benefits of mindfulness and awareness. A man had gone camping with some friends and pulled into the campground in the middle of the afternoon. It was crowded and noisy; kids were running around, dogs were barking, and people were yelling. Later that night, after everyone had gone to sleep, the man woke to check on a sound he heard, and as he stood outside his camper, he heard water running in a small creek not 10 feet from where he stood. During the day, with all the commotion, not only had he not heard the stream, he didn't even know it existed.

"In many ways our minds are like the noisy campground: so filled with the distractions of the everyday world that we are unable to detect beauty and stillness of a gentle creek that is so close to us.

"When we learn to clear away the clutter and still the chatter, we will be able to find the beauty and stillness of the mind."

—*Eric B. Robins, M.D.*

SINGLE-POINT CONCENTRATION, SIMULTANEOUS AWARENESS, AND EXPANDED AWARENESS

As you become more proficient with the Mindfulness Meditation, you may wish to hold your awareness on two and then all three of the focal points simultaneously throughout the meditation. This helps you move from single-point concentration to *expanded awareness*, the ability to be aware of many things at the same time. Expanded awareness is the ultimate goal of high-level meditation for it leads to what some call *cosmic consciousness*, a state in which the barriers between subject (meditator) and object (the world), between knower and known melt away. It is true oneness. The conscious mind can focus on only one thing at a time, but the unconscious mind, when it establishes contact with the higher self during periods of prolonged stillness, is capable of focusing on many things at once.

You have already received some elementary training in simultaneous awareness. In scanning, you learn to be aware of your breathing, your scanning target, and the sensitivity of your hand chakra. In projecting prana, you have to be concerned with your breathing, your source chakra, your projecting chakra, and your target. And in the illumination technique in the Meditation on Twin Hearts, you are instructed to be aware of your chanting, the light on your crown, the inner stillness, and the gap between the OMs. These all help you build expanded awareness. The progression from one to two to three focal points in the Mindfulness Meditation will give you a more formal practice path should you desire to work more purposefully on expanded awareness.

You need not try for expanded awareness to get the physical health benefits of the Mindfulness Meditation. The multiple focus is offered for those who are interested in the higher-level and more spiritual aspects of meditation.

MEDITATION ON TWIN HEARTS

Of all the techniques developed and taught by Grandmaster Choa Kok Sui, perhaps none prompts as many glowing testimonials of personal healing and positive life transformation as the Meditation on Twin Hearts. This meditation is truly special. It works on the physical, mental, and spiritual levels to open the heart chakra (the physical heart) and the crown chakra (the spiritual heart), thereby enabling you to draw down a great amount of high-quality divine energy into the crown. The prana that this meditation produces greatly promotes physical and mental health as well as inner illumination.

An energetically dirty aura, one that is clogged with unreconciled negative emotions, anxieties, anger, and fears, appears as a shimmering white cloud filled with dark-colored smudges and small vortices. These smudges and vortices are energetic disturbances that form functional boundaries in your energy body. They block the smooth, plentiful flow of prana and lead to physical ailments.

When someone who can see auras observes a person practicing the Meditation on Twin Hearts, he sees a great downpouring of brilliant white light rushing into the crown and spreading throughout the entire energy body. This divine prana purges the energy body of contamination, which is how Meditation on Twin Hearts produces physical healing.

This opening of the crown and the increased flow of divine energy also makes possible inner illumination. After blessing the earth with the spiritual energy, you meditate on OM and the gap or the stillness between the OMs for about 10 minutes. You then let go and extend that period of stillness. Meditating on the gap between the OMs and during the extended period of stillness enables you to make contact with your higher self or soul. Repeated prolonged stillness and contact with your soul produces that state of inner illumination.

Here are just a few stories of people who have experienced a positive impact in their lives from practicing the Meditation on Twin Hearts:

As a school administrator, I mediate stressful and negative situations among students, parents, and coworkers. By practicing the Meditation on Twin Hearts, I am able to resolve conflicts and respond in a more calm and compassionate manner. I utilize positive thoughts and emotions to find solutions in a constructive way.

—SANDRA WASHINGTON, LOS ANGELES

The Meditation on Twin Hearts has made a profound impact on my life in the last two years since I started regular meditation. It has increased my healing ability, and changed the way I view life and my purpose in life. . . . The Meditation on Twin Hearts is my daily opportunity to become a true channel of needed blessings to all people.

—MARK WIECZOREK, REGO PARK, NEW YORK

I have been using the Meditation on Twin Hearts since 1996. [As a result, I have had] less stress, a more centered and compassionate outlook, and better overall health. I am a substance abuse counselor and have been able to utilize this meditation in my work. [I have noted] significant positive effects in [my clients'] progress. Only a brief period of time listening to the guided meditation leaves one feeling centered, energized, and serene.

—MOSES MCCLUSKEY, LOS ANGELES

Before Performing the Meditation on Twin Hearts

Since you're working with prana of greater quantity and higher quality in the Meditation on Twin Hearts, you need to be aware of certain aspects of the meditation, as well as several contraindications:

- People with high blood pressure, heart ailments, and glaucoma should not perform Meditation on Twin Hearts. This meditation generates tremendous energy and may aggravate those conditions.

- People under the age of 18 should not practice the illumination technique (Step 7 of the meditation) because their bodies are not fully mature and are unable to tolerate the energy this meditation produces.

- Before you do this meditation, pay close attention to the energetic cleanliness of your meditation environment. A dirty room may cancel out the effect of the meditation, or even contaminate you as you meditate. Refer to the techniques for cleaning your environment in Chapter 10.

- Make sure you do a full 5 minutes of physical exercise before and after meditating to avoid energetic congestion. We recommend that both routines include at least one set of Cleansing Physical Exercises (Exercise 10-I), since they were specifically designed to open the body's energetic channels and spread around the energy.

- Perform the blessings with real feeling, not mechanically. Feel and concentrate on the feelings of love you conjure up as you bless the earth. Add visualization, if you wish. See a golden-pinkish light emitting from your hands and bathing the earth. See people's faces smiling with peace, love, and joy. See nations that are in conflict laying down their weapons. See people living together in harmony and actually performing good deeds for one another.

EXERCISE 11–B: *Meditation on Twin Hearts*

You can either follow the steps presented below for this meditation or use the Meditation on Twin Hearts CD prepared by Grandmaster Choa Kok Sui (see "For More Information on Pranic Healing Products and Classes" section). Begin with steps 1 through 4 from the Mindfulness Meditation, but leave out the body relaxation sequence. Proceed.

1. Invoke. Close your eyes, bow your head, and raise your hands a few inches off your lap. Turn your palms upward. If you haven't been using an invocation, here is one that you can use:

   To the divine Father and Mother, I humbly ask for your divine blessing,
   guidance, protection, help, and illumination. With thanks and in full faith.

2. Perform several cycles of pranic breathing.
3. Activate your heart chakra. Press your heart chakra with one finger for a moment or

two, then place your hands back on your lap. Conjure up feelings of love and sweetness. Really feel the feelings of love and compassion welling up inside of you. This is easily done by simply recalling a few happy events in your life, or imagining the face of someone you love very dearly in front of you and reexperiencing the loving feelings you have toward them. Smile inwardly at your heart chakra. This takes about 2 minutes.

4. Activate your crown chakra. Tap your crown chakra with a finger, then place your hand back on your lap. Imagine another scene where you feel the feelings of love and sweetness. Really feel the feelings of love and compassion welling up inside of you. Smile inwardly at your crown chakra. This takes about 2 minutes.

5. Bless the earth with lovingkindness through your heart chakra. Stay aware of those feelings of love and sweetness and raise your hands to chest level with your palms facing outward. Imagine the earth in front of you about the size of a small ball. Be aware of your heart and your hand chakras as you bless the earth (Figure 11–1). (*Note:* You can

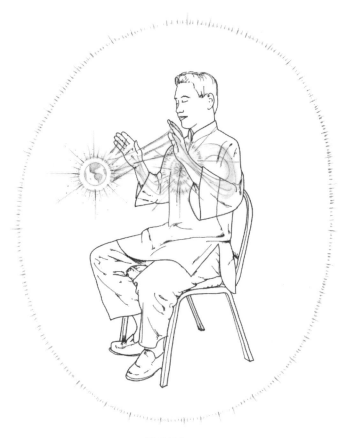

FIGURE 11–1

bless the earth with a prayer or language of your own choosing, however, we include a sample here.) Recite the first stanza of the Prayer of St. Francis of Assisi:

Lord, make me an instrument of your peace, . . .

Feel the divine peace within your heart flow to your hands and outward to the earth. Bless the earth for a minute or so. See the beautiful pink light of blessings flow from your heart to your hand to the earth.

Where there is hatred, let me sow love, . . .

Feel divine love well up within your heart and flow to your hands and outward to the earth. Bless the earth for a minute or so.

Where there is injury, pardon, . . .

Bless the earth with divine forgiveness. Bless areas of the earth where there is conflict. See the conflicts resolved.

Where there is doubt, faith; where there is despair, hope, . . .

Bless the earth with hope and faith. Bless people who are having a difficult time.

Where there is darkness, light; where there is sadness, joy, . . .

Bless the earth with light and joy. Bless areas and countries where there is strife.

6. Now bless the earth with lovingkindness through your crown chakra. Be aware of your crown chakra as you continue to bless the earth (Figure 11–2). See the beautiful golden light of blessings flow from your crown to your hand and through your hands to the earth.

Let the entire earth, let every person and every being be blessed with lovingkindness, ...
with sweetness, . . . with joy and with happiness, . . .

Continue blessing the earth for a minute. See every person filled with love and joy.

7. Now bless the earth with lovingkindness through both your heart and your crown chakra simultaneously. Be aware of both your heart and your crown chakra as you continue to bless the earth. See the beautiful golden light of blessings flow from your crown and your heart to your hands and through your hands to the earth (Figure 11–3).

From the Heart of God, let every person, every sentient being be blessed
with lovingkindness, . . .

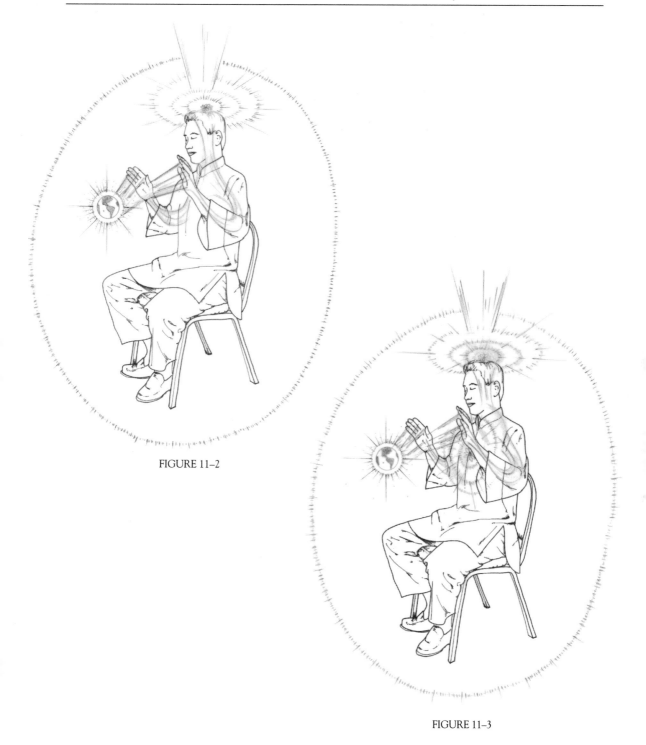

FIGURE 11–2

FIGURE 11–3

Continue blessing the earth and seeing every person filled with love, joy, and peace.

Let every person, every being be blessed with great joy, happiness, and divine inner peace, . . .

See people with their hearts filled with joy, faith, and hope. See the expression on their faces.

Let every person, every being be blessed with understanding, with harmony, with good will, and with the will to do good. . . .

See people actually doing good for other people.

8. Illumination technique. Put your hands back into your lap, palms up. Visualize a brilliant point of dazzling golden light just above your crown (Figure 11–4). See it clearly

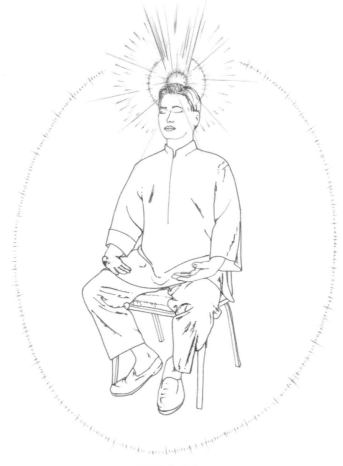

FIGURE 11–4

as if it were a focused point of sunlight reflecting off newly fallen snow. After you have locked in the image, begin silently chanting to yourself the mantra OM. Pronounce it silently to yourself slowly and purposefully: "OOOMMMM . . . " Breathe deeply and slowly as you chant. Gently put your awareness on the point of light above your head, the OM, and the gap between the OMs for 5 to 10 minutes. Then stop the mantra, stop visualizing the point of light, and simply let go for a few minutes. Let your mind go blank and extend the sense of inner peace and stillness. Do this for about 5 minutes, though as you progress, you can stretch this out for as long as you like. If thoughts or external noises intrude, note them without reacting and bring your attention back to the stillness.

9. Release the excess energy. The surplus of energy this meditation generates must be dispersed in order to avoid congestion. You could project the energy outward but why not use it for additional positive effect? Thus, bless the earth again. Raise your hands to the blessing position and simply bless the earth with light and love. You may wish to visualize the beams of golden-pink light leaving your hand and caressing the earth in front of you. You may also bless your family, loved ones, friends, home, job, and any other personal project you're working on. Do this for about 30 seconds. Then return your hands to your lap.

10. Grounding. Use the same grounding routine that you used in the Mindfulness Meditation.

11. End the meditation by giving thanks. A variation of the invocation is one way to do this. Simply raise your hands to the same invocation posture and say:

> *To the divine Father and Mother, I humbly give you thanks for your divine blessing, guidance, protection, help, and illumination. With thanks and in full faith.*

12. Repeat cleansing physical exercises.

A Few Final Notes on Meditation

•   Your outlook during meditation should be positive and expectant but neutral. Don't focus on or expect results. For example, in the Meditation on Twin Hearts, illumination rarely comes during a first session, though you begin accruing the benefits of greater energy and health immediately. Approach it as a climber approaches a mountain: He's aware of the peak and expects to get there, yet he doesn't focus on it. He looks only to the next handhold or foothold.

•   Some people experience shaking or strong emotions welling up within them. As indicated earlier, meditation is an indirect clearing technique, and trembling or sudden feelings are evidence of energetic blockages being cleared out and the emotions associated with those blockages being released. If you encounter any discomfort during meditation, respond according to your personal threshold. Some people breathe more deeply and continue with the meditation. If you wish, however, you can stop the session and sweep and clean the area where you feel discomfort. You can meditate later.

- Both meditations should take about 20 minutes. In the Meditation on Twin Hearts, that includes about 10 minutes for blessing the earth and 10 minutes for illumination. As you gain experience, you may spend more time on the illumination portion.

- Beginners may experience slight congestion in the chest or heart area as they bless the earth during the Meditation on Twin Hearts. If this is uncomfortable, simply sweep and clean the area after you are finished. If it gets too uncomfortable, stop your meditation, and sweep and clean the area. You can meditate later or the next day.

- When you are able to hold simultaneous awareness on the point of light and the gap in the Meditation on Twin Hearts, you may experience an inner explosion of light. This is normal, though it can be startling at first. Again, respond according to your own personal comfort threshold. If you can, simply breathe deeply and feel the feeling of the experience. If you need to, stop meditating and close with giving thanks, then perform grounding.

FREQUENCY OF MEDITATION PRACTICE

Meditation is best practiced daily, and daily practice obviously offers the quickest progress. But daily practice may not always be feasible, given your other commitments. You still get excellent energetic and health benefits from meditating three to five times a week. Here are three different meditation schedules for you to consider, depending on the time you have available:

Most Frequent Practice:

Meditation on Twin Hearts in the morning, and Mindfulness Meditation in the evening. Or, Mindfulness in the morning and Meditation on Twin Hearts in the evening.

Daily Practice:

Alternate meditations daily: Meditation on Twin Hearts one day, then Mindfulness Meditation the next.

Moderate Practice:

Meditate three to five times per week: Meditation on Twin Hearts on two to three days; Mindfulness Meditation on the others.

MEDITATION CHECKLIST

Mindfulness Meditation

1. Do physical exercises, either cleansing physical exercises or exercises of your own choosing.
2. Be seated in a cool, dark room; place your hands palms up in your lap.
3. Put your tongue on your palate.
4. Invoke.
5. Do 10 cycles of pranic breathing.
6. Do progressive physical relaxation.
7. Determine the point of focus and stay with it; add a second and then a third point of focus, if you wish and as you progress.
8. Do periodic posture checks.
9. Begin with 10 minutes of awareness, building up to 20 or 30.
10. Ground.
11. Get up and do cleansing physical exercises.

Meditation on Twin Hearts

(*Note:* The Grandmaster Choa Kok Sui meditation CD takes you through all these steps.)

1. Do physical exercises, either cleansing physical exercises or exercises of your own choosing.
2. Be seated in a cool, dark room; place your hands palms up in your lap.
3. Put your tongue on your palate.
4. Invoke.
5. Do 10 cycles of pranic breathing.
6. Do progressive physical relaxation (optional).
7. Activate the heart chakra.
8. Activate the crown chakra.
9. Bless the earth with lovingkindness through the heart chakra.

10. Bless the earth with lovingkindness through the crown chakra.
11. Bless the earth with lovingkindness through the heart and crown chakras simultaneously.
12. Do the Illumination technique.
13. Release your excess energy by blessing the earth again.
14. Ground.
15. End with an invocation, giving thanks.
16. Get up and do cleansing physical exercises.

Meditation is the catalyst for your energetic self-healing. It cleanses your body and mind and makes them more able to accept greater quantities and higher qualities of healing prana. The experience of New York Pranic Healing student Cynthia de Leon is typical: After getting hit by a car and suffering a fractured fibula and several gashes on her right leg, she endured constant pain, which could not be addressed with medication or pain-killers because she was allergic to them. At the same time, she was going through emotional upheavals brought about by a pending divorce. She said, "The daily practice of Meditation of Twin Hearts and Pranic Healing eased tremendously the physical and emotional trauma that I was going through. It allowed me to function properly and even perform outstandingly in various areas of my life with great facility. . . . " It was her meditation practice that gave her peace of mind to endure her hardships, and also the ability to draw in greater quantities of healing energy to perform regular self-healings.

SIX STEPS DAILY PRACTICE ROUTINE—UPDATE

You may practice meditation by itself or incorporate it into your existing morning or evening routine. Here's a suggested sequence:

1. Invoke for guidance and protection.
2. Cut cords.
3. Do cleansing physical exercises.
4. Do pranic breathing.
5. Do direct clearing techniques, as needed.
6. Meditation (alternate Mindfulness Meditation with Meditation on Twin Hearts, according to your schedule and preference).
7. Do cleansing physical exercises after meditation.

8. Do standard warm-up.
9. Do hand sensitivity, scanning, sweeping, energizing practice.
10. Do special exercises: general self-sweeping, general stress-reduction, work/house cleaning, and so forth.

Add the other elements of energetic hygiene to your daily routine as you are able, or as you see fit.

In the next chapter, you'll learn to really turn up the voltage with the sixth and final step to self-healing, two powerful *energy-generation* routines: Mentalphysics Exercises and a unique Pranic Healing version of Tibetan Yogic Exercises and the Metaphysical Exercises.

CHAPTER 12

Plugging In, Charging Up— Two Powerful Energy-Generation Exercises

"Before I learned the Tibetan Yogic Exercises and the Mentalphysics Exercises, I was constantly fatigued. As I look back on my life now, I realize my energy level was always below average. As a teen and in my twenties, I tired easily, and my sex drive was not what it should have been for a young man at that age. As I took on the pressures of being a husband, a father, a physician, and a surgeon, I found my energy level even more difficult to maintain. After I learned the Tibetan Yogic Exercises and the Mentalphysics Exercises and began to practice them regularly, my energy level exploded. They literally changed my life. I cannot recommend these energy-generating exercises highly enough."

—ERIC B. ROBINS, M.D.

The last of the six steps to self-healing is a pair of energy-generation exercises that are the crown jewels of such exercises. The first is called the Tibetan Yogic Exercises, though it is also known as the Rejuvenation Rite. The second is called the Mentalphysics Exercises.

There are better-known energy-generating exercises, including some forms of yoga, different types of breathwork, *chi kung*, and tai chi. But none offers the rapid prana-generating potential, or are as easy to perform as the Tibetan Yogic Exercises and Mentalphysics Exercises. This isn't to say, though, that the Tibetan Yogic Exercises and Mentalphysics Exercises are completely unknown. Both are practiced by people today, though knowledge of the Tibetan Yogic Exercises is more widespread. What *isn't* known, however, is exactly why these exercises are so effective. Very few people—and virtually no one aside from those who have taken a special class from Grandmaster Choa Kok Sui—know that a series of simple modifications makes these routines even more powerful, easier, and quicker to perform.

Both the Tibetan Yogic Exercises and the Mentalphysics Exercises are part of that larger body of ancient esoteric root teachings that spiritual masters and teachers throughout history, such as Grandmaster Choa Kok Sui, have passed on to their students. They are a powerful addition to your health routine because they drive prana from the lower chakras to the upper chakras, distributing this energy more easily throughout the body and helping regenerate it. The Tibetan Yogic Exercises have the added benefits of drawing down tremendous amounts of spiritual energy and physicalizing it into the body, as well opening the body's two main prana pumping stations: the neck and the lower back.

Even though these exercises build upon pranic breathing, we present them to students *after* they learn pranic breathing because they both are higher-level practices that generate a lot of energy. As one practitioner reports, "After doing the Mentalphysics Exercises, my physical, emotional, mental, and spiritual bodies are rejuvenated and energetically charged with clean, fresh energy. I feel balanced and am experiencing a more positive outlook on life." Another practitioner offers that, after performing the Tibetan Yogic Exercises, "It's like my gas tank was empty, and I just filled it up." A third explains that she understands the true benefits of these energy-generating exercises particularly when she *doesn't* do them. "If I miss doing them for only one day I notice a lack of energy and 'mental scatteredness,'" she says.

The Tibetan Yogic Exercises

The Tibetan Yogic Exercises are five simple postures whose benefits include greater overall energy, increased or recovered sex drive, weight loss, and even regeneration of hair. Grandmaster Choa Kok Sui taught them to his private students for years, but they've been popularized through several recent books, *The Five Tibetans,* by Christopher S. Kilham; and *The Five Rites of Rejuvenation* by Peter Kelder, the original book that introduced the exercises to the Western public, which was then reissued under the title *Ancient Secrets of the Fountain of Youth,* to which Kilham gives credit. Kelder learned the routine from a retired British army officer who had been taught them by a group of Tibetan monks in the Himalayas. There are Chinese and Indian versions of these exercises as well, but the Tibetan form is presented here because it is the easiest to perform while still retaining great energetic potency—especially with Grandmaster Choa Kok Sui's modifications.

Mentalphysics Exercises

The Mentalphysics routine is a set of breathing exercises originally developed by Edwin J. Dingle, an esoteric scholar and cartographer who lived and studied in China and Tibet in the early part of this century. While on an expedition in the mountains of Tibet, he was robbed and then attacked by wild animals and left for dead in the wilderness. A Tibetan lama saved his life with herbs and energy healing. The lama also gave him a secret set of exercises to nurse him back to health, which Dingle introduced to his students as the Mentalphysics Exercises. The original exercises by themselves are quite powerful and enable practitioners to increase their general prana supply substantially. The original routine is also quite lengthy: up to 49 breaths that take a full hour. The modified Mentalphysics Exercises presented here can be performed in less than 9 minutes with a 10-fold increase in power.

The Power of the Mentalphysics Exercises

"When I first went to teach Pranic Healing in Chicago a few years ago, I was informed that there would be a 92-year-old woman attending the class. I was concerned that she might not be strong enough to do all the practices for two full days. Two local workshop organizers laughed and said, 'She can walk around the block faster than most 30-year-olds!' Then they told me the woman's story. Laura Appelgren was diagnosed with breast cancer five decades ago. Her doctors in Wisconsin, where she lived at the time, wanted to perform a mastectomy immediately. She declined. Shortly thereafter she read an ad in a magazine that said, 'Knowledge is power. Come and learn to breathe in the desert.' It was an ad for the Institute of Mentalphysics. Against her husband's wishes, she took a train and 'learned to breathe' in the desert for a week with Edwin J. Dingle. After practicing the exercises for a while, her cancer was completely gone. She continued the exercises for the next 50 years.

"I had Laura lead the class in the Mentalphysics Exercises. Most of the class, which was much younger than Laura, couldn't keep up with her pace.

"At the time of her passing—in her sleep, peacefully—Laura still had all her teeth, and didn't need glasses or hearing aids."

—*Master Stephen Co*

ENERGY-GENERATING TIPS

These tips apply to both the Tibetan Yogic Exercises and the Mentalphysics Exercises.

1. Perform the exercises in an open area with good ventilation. Performing them outside is ideal (but not in the sun; the solar prana is too strong). If you're doing them indoors, keep the windows open to allow fresh air in.

2. For comfort, wear loose clothing, and perform the exercises on an empty stomach.

3. Shower or bathe before practicing these exercises, not after; water washes away prana.

4. The optimum time for performing these exercises is following meditation, especially in the morning. After you meditate, perform your postmeditation grounding routine and exercises. Then perform either the Tibetan Yogic Exercises or the Mentalphysics Exercises.

5. Practice good energetic hygiene. Beginners typically have energy bodies that are dirty and unaccustomed to handling as much prana as these exercises generate. Before you begin your practice of the Tibetan Yogic Exercises and Mentalphysics Exercises, review the energetic hygiene routine at the end of Chapter 10. At minimum, do the following:
   - Keep your diet clean and healthy.
   - Keep your meditation and energy-generation practice area clean; clean it at least once a week with with Exercise 10–J.
   - Perform the Cleansing Physical Exercises and pranic breathing daily.
   - Take a salt bath two or three times a week.

6. It's best not to practice these exercises in the evening, at least until you see how you react to them. Because they produce a lot of energy, you might have difficulty falling asleep.

7. If the exercises produce physical discomfort, discontinue them until you speak to your physician. As noted, the exercises are simple to perform, but every person has an individual threshold for activity and discomfort. If you have any physical problems before performing them or experience discomfort during the exercises, stop and consult your physician.

8. If you feel jittery or overenergized, stop and take a break. Don't go any further in your practice. Perform general sweeping to clear away the excess prana, and take a salt bath if necessary. Resume practice after your energy condition is stabilized.

9. Pick one of the two routines and become proficient with that one before going on to the other. Don't jump into performing both the Tibetan Yogic Exercises and the Mentalphysics Exercises at the same time. Try both routines to see which feels better for you and to get the coordination of the movements down. But choose one or the other as

you begin to practice in earnest. After you become comfortable with one exercise, incorporate the other into your daily routine.

10. You can begin performing either one of these exercises as a full routine immediately. With the modified versions presented here, there is no need to build up gradually. If, however, any movement or breathing exercise causes you discomfort, you may wish to perform a shortened routine and build up to the full routine. Of course, with any discomfort, it is also wise to check with your physician before continuing.

11. Many people like to perform the Tibetan Yogic Exercises or Mentalphysics Exercises after their postmeditation exercises. Meditation provides a good energetic warm-up, and the Cleansing Physical Exercises provide a good physical warm-up before beginning these powerful energy-generation routines. If, however, you are performing either of these routines on their own, we advise that you stretch for about 5 minutes to loosen your joints and use the Cleansing Physical Exercises.

12. Students often inquire whether they can practice the "original" or unmodified Tibetan Yogic Exercises and Mentalphysics Exercises. Absolutely. For the books that include them see the "For Further Reference" section. Our experience has been, however, that once students practice both the original and modified versions of both exercises, they find that the modified exercises generate more prana and are easier to perform. The modified routines presented here also take much less time. In the case of the Tibetan Yogic Exercises, you only need to perform each of the five exercises a maximum of nine times, versus 21 times in the original version. In the case of the Mentalphysics Exercises, you only need to perform each of the six main exercises (3 through 9) once, versus seven times in the original version.

EXERCISE 12-A: *The Tibetan Yogic Exercises*

Key modification for all the Tibetan Yogic Exercises: Place your tongue on your palate before you begin and keep it there throughout the exercises. This connects the main energy channels in your energy body and promotes greater flow of prana throughout the body.

The First Tibetan Yogic Exercise

Starting position: Stand erect with arms outstretched comfortably and horizontal to the floor. Keep your fingers together and your palms downward (Photo 12–a).

Exercise: Turn clockwise (to your right) at a measured pace for nine revolutions. Inhale through the nose during the first spin, hold it while you spin until you have a full breath, and then hold the breath until you've completed spinning. Then exhale through either your mouth or nose. Try to hold your breath for the entire nine spins. But if this is difficult at first, simply hold it for as many revolutions as you can and build up to holding it for the full nine turns. As you progress, you should increase the speed of your revolutions, but let your sense of equilibrium guide your progress. Never spin so rapidly that you get dizzy. (*Note:* If you do get dizzy, however, most people find that continuing immediately to the other exercises relieves the dizziness.) If nine revolutions is difficult for you, begin slowly with a fewer number and build up to nine revolutions. After you complete the exercise, stand up, perform two cycles of pranic breathing, and be aware of your entire body.

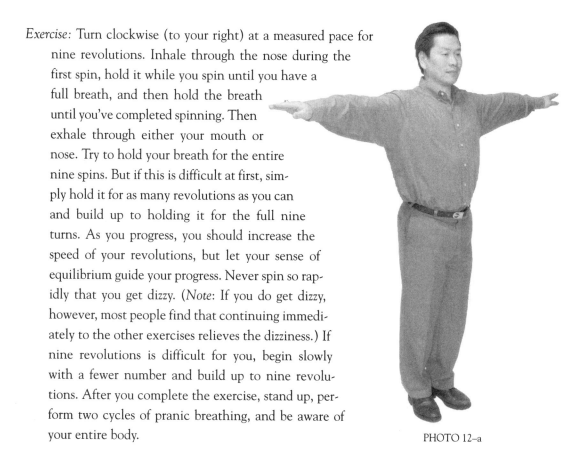

PHOTO 12–a

Key modification: The breathing, which you may recognize as a form of extended rhythm and retention. It adds exceptional power to a simple movement.

Energetic effect: This exercise draws down tremendous amounts of spiritual energy. You can scan your crown before and after spinning and notice a great increase in size and strength.

The Second Tibetan Yogic Exercise

Starting position: Lie flat on the floor, face up. Pull your legs up toward you until your knees are at a 45-degree angle, while keeping your feet still flat on the floor. You may wish to lie on a rug or mat, but don't do this exercise on a bed because it doesn't offer sufficient support for your back. Fully extend your arms along your sides, and place the palms of your hands against the floor. Keep your fingers close together.

Exercise: In one simultaneous movement, bend your neck to raise your head off the floor and tuck your chin against your chest, while lifting your legs gently into an abs-crunch position (Photo 12–b). Then slowly lower both the head and the feet to the floor. Breathe in deeply through your nose as you lift your legs, hold your breath for a few seconds at the top position, and then breathe out through either your nose or mouth as you lower your legs. Perform nine times total. After you complete the exercise, stand up, perform two cycles of pranic breathing, and be aware of your entire body.

Key modifications: The breathing, which utilizes rhythm and retention. Also, the original exercise calls for a straight-leg leg lift, which can create strain on the lower back. The modified movement here is easier to perform but still maintains, due to breath retention, great energy-generating ability.

Energetic effect: This exercise physicalizes the spiritual energy drawn down by the First Tibetan Yogic Exercise in the throat and sex chakras, the centers of creativity. It also increases your sexual energy.

The Third Tibetan Yogic Exercise

Starting position: Kneel on the floor with your spine straight. Tuck your chin against your chest (Photo 12–c).

Exercise: Begin your inhale through your nostrils, and as you do so, raise your head up and back as far as it can comfortably go. Don't strain. Time your inhale so that as your lungs are full, your head is all the way back (Photo 12–d). Exhale through the mouth and move your head back to the starting position. Your exhale should be forceful and audible but keep your face and cheeks relaxed. Exhale strongly with a *shu* sound. Your cheeks should puff out a bit and you should hear your breath rushing out as you exhale. Time your exhale so that, as your lungs empty, your head has returned to the starting position. Initially, the outbreath may move your tongue off the roof of your mouth, but with practice, you can keep it there. Perform nine times total. After you complete the exercise, stand up, perform two cycles of pranic breathing, and be aware of your entire body.

Key modifications: There are several. First, the breathing pattern—which is called "Rapid Turtle Breathing" in Chinese esoteric systems (and the "Memory-Development Breath" in the Mentalphysics Exercises later in the chapter)—generates a tremendous amount

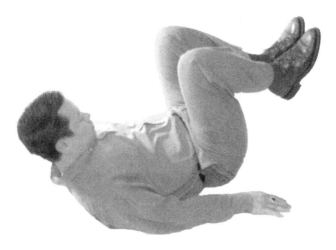

PHOTO 12–b

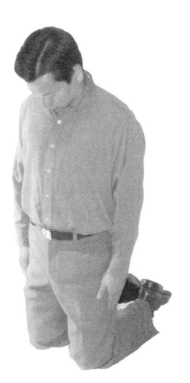

PHOTO 12–c

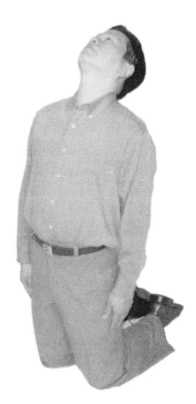

PHOTO 12–d

of prana. Second, the *shu* exhalation, which is one of the Taoist "healing sounds" magnifies the overall energy-generating effect. Third, the original exercise calls for hyperextending the back and neck from the kneeling position, which can place strain on the spine. This modified movement is easier to perform and just as powerful.

Energetic effect: This exercise cleanses the head chakras and circulates energy through the throat and sex chakras. It also enhances mental clarity.

The Fourth Tibetan Yogic Exercise

Starting position: Sit on the floor with your knees at a 45-degree angle and your feet flat on the floor and about 12 inches apart. With the trunk of the body erect and perpendicular to the ground, place the palms of your hands on the floor alongside the buttocks. Tuck the chin forward against the chest (Photo 12–e).

Exercise: Simultaneously move your head backward as far as it will go comfortably while raising your body by bending the knees and pushing off the ground with your feet. The knees bend while the arms remain straight. The position you are assuming is roughly a table, with the head pointing downward, the trunk of the body parallel to the ground,

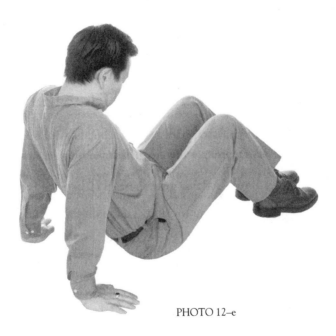

PHOTO 12–e

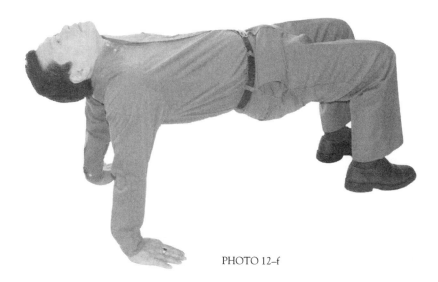

PHOTO 12–f

and the lower legs perpendicular to the ground (Photo 12–f). Breathe out as you move up into the table position, then tense every muscle in your body for a few seconds in that position. Breathe in as you gently lower yourself to the ground. Perform this nine times total. After you complete the exercise, stand up, perform two cycles of pranic breathing, and be aware of your entire body.

Key modifications: There are several. First, the breathing pattern, which is the opposite of what you might expect, generates much more energy in this posture. Second, the tension adds to your prana-generating capability. Third, the original exercise calls for you to begin with legs straight and to move the body upward by pushing the feet flat to the floor. The modified version puts less stress on the shoulders and knees, but it is just as powerful.

Energetic effect: This exercise cleanses the entire body and distributes the prana to the extremities.

The Fifth Tibetan Yogic Exercise

Starting position: Begin in a woman's push-up position, with the hands flat on the floor directly below or up to 1 foot in front of the shoulders, and the knees and shins flat on the floor. Pull your head slightly back but do not strain (Photo 12–g).

Exercise: In one simultaneous movement, move your hips up and back, while pivoting your head downward, bending your elbows slightly, and breathing in through your nose. Your knees, shins, and feet stay in the starting position (Photo 12–h). Then bring the hips down to their original position, straighten your elbows, and pull your head back, exhaling through the nose or mouth as you do so. Perform nine times total. After you complete the exercise, stand up, perform two cycles of pranic breathing, and be aware of your entire body.

Key modifications: There are two important modifications. First, the original version calls for you to use two hatha yoga positions, the "cobra," to begin, and the "downward dog," to end. This movement is similar to an exaggerated push-up and requires some degree of strength, flexibility, and coordination. The modified version is much less difficult to perform but still very powerful. Second, as in the modified Fourth Tibetan Yogic Exercise, the breathing pattern here is reversed—breathing in as you move down and out as you move up. Experiments show that this distributes the energy throughout the body much more effectively.

Energetic effect: This exercise circulates and balances the energy in the front and back meridians of the body. It also helps move prana from the lower to the upper chakras.

After you complete the exercises, simply walk around and stretch a bit and resume your daily activities.

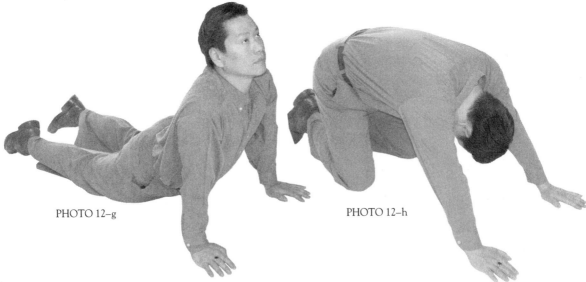

PHOTO 12–g   PHOTO 12–h

> ## Modified Tibetans Are Easier on the Body
>
> "The modified Tibetan Yogic Exercises are remarkable not only for their energy-generating capability, but also because they can be practiced even by those who are physically restricted. I've shown them to numerous patients who reported feeling run-down and were unable to perform the original version because of joint pain, arthritis, weight problems, or lack of flexibility and strength. Nearly all are able to perform the modified Tibetan Yogic Exercises and feel the energetic benefits very quickly."
>
> —*Eric B. Robins, M.D.*

EXERCISE 12–B: *Mentalphysics Exercises*

You can perform the first two breaths either standing or seated. Stand for the rest. Keep your feet flat on the floor and your spine straight throughout.

Key modification for all Mentalphysics Exercises: Place your tongue on your palate before you begin and keep it there throughout the exercises.

The First Mentalphysics Exercise: The Harmonic Breath (also known as Balancing Breathing)

Starting position: (*Note:* Wash your hands with salt soap or spray them with alcohol before beginning this exercise. Your hands can pick up a lot of dirty energy.) Raise your left hand and rest your left thumb lightly against your left nostril. Keep the other fingers of your left hand relaxed (Photo 12–i).

Exercise: Exhale comfortably. Pinch your left nostril shut with your left thumb, and inhale for a six count through your right nostril. (One second per count is a good pace.) Pinch your right nostril shut with your left forefinger, and hold for a count of three. Take your left thumb off your left nostril, and exhale for a count of six through the left nostril. Pinch your left nostril again, and hold for a count of three. Open your left nostril, and keeping your right nostril pinched shut, inhale for a count of six through your left nostril. Then pinch your

PHOTO 12–i

left nostril shut with your left thumb, and hold for a count of three. Take your left forefinger off your right nostril and exhale for a count of six. Close the right nostril off again, and hold for a count of three. This constitutes one cycle. Repeat the sequence four more times for a total of five breaths. When you are finished, perform one cycle of pranic breathing, and then relax and be aware of your body for a few moments.

Key modification: The original Mentalphysics program calls for this rhythm: inhale for four counts, hold for 16, exhale for eight; then again with the other nostril, inhale for four, hold for 16, exhale for eight. The 6–3–6–3 sequence is the optimum rhythm and retention sequence.

Energetic effect: This exercise cleans and balances the energy of both sides of the brain. It also cleans and balances the energy of the left and right sides of the body.

A *few notes on the Harmonic Breath/Balancing Breathing:*

- The 6–3–6–3 sequence is the optimal breathing pattern. If you find it difficult to hold your breath for three counts, you can do the 7–1–7–1 sequence.
- If one of your nostrils is clogged, try this: Several minutes before the exercise, roll up a towel or magazine into a tight cylinder and place it firmly into the armpit opposite the clogged nostril. If your right nostril is clogged, place the rolled-up towel under your left armpit. This puts pressure on a key meridian that energizes your nasal passages and should clear up your congestion.

The Second Mentalphysics Exercise: The Memory-Developing Breath (also known as Rapid Turtle Breathing)

Starting position: It's the same as for the third Tibetan Yogic Exercise, except that you can stand or sit. (Photo 12–j)

Exercise: The breathing pattern is exactly the same as for the third Tibetan Yogic Exercise. As with that exercise, time your inhales so that as your lungs are full, your head is all the way back.

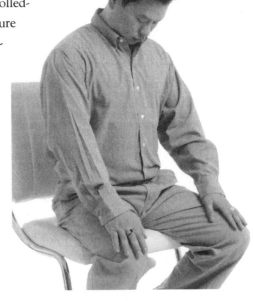

PHOTO 12–j

Then time your exhales so that, as your lungs empty, your head has returned to the starting position. Perform one set of 14 cycles of Rapid Turtle Breathing. Pause for a moment. Then do a second set of 14 breaths, then take a break. Then do a third set of 14 breaths, then take a break. Finally, do a fourth set of *seven* breaths. (Caution: If at any time you get dizzy, slow down. Take a break and walk around. You should inhale and exhale briskly, but you shouldn't hyperventilate.) When you are finished, perform one cycle of pranic breathing and then relax and be aware of your body for a few moments.

Key modification: It's the rhythm. The original Mentalphysics program calls for the rhythm to be seven sets of seven-count breaths. But the 14–14–14–7 rhythm is more powerful.

Energetic effect: This exercise is a forced cleansing of the energy channels. It cleans and energizes the head and the spinal column all the way down to the basic chakra. The vigorous head movement pulls the energy up and down your spine.

The Third Mentalphysics Exercise: The Revitalizing Breath

Starting position: Perform this and the following six exercises while standing. Begin in an erect posture. Keep your feet and ankles together, your spine and neck straight, and your head facing forward. Your arms are straight down with hands at your side. Keep your fingers together. Keep your mouth closed and your teeth lightly touching (Photo 12–k).

Exercise: Exhale audibly through your mouth until your lungs are empty. Then inhale deeply, completely filling your lungs. After you fill your lungs, take one final sniff through the nose, and then lock in the breath by tensing all the muscles of your body. Tense your neck, clench your jaw, straighten out your arms and legs, and tighten your torso and buttocks. Squeeze and tense, but don't strain. Most important, squeeze your pubococcygeal or PC muscle. This is the muscle group that runs from the pubic area through the perineum and back to the anus. It controls your urinary and bowel movement functions. Thus, when you contract

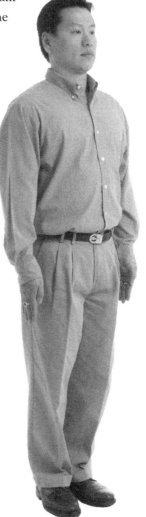

PHOTO 12–k

the PC muscle, it is as if you were trying to prevent yourself from going to the bathroom; you're "holding it," both front and back. For women, squeezing the front portion of the PC muscle is the same as Kegel exercises. Hold your breath and this bodily tension for 5 seconds. Exhale, then release the bodily tension. Perform one cycle of pranic breathing and then relax and be aware of your body for a few moments.

Key modification for Third through Ninth Mentalphysics Exercises: Squeezing the PC muscle. The original Mentalphysics program omits this entirely and suggests you begin holding each breath for 20 to 30 seconds and then gradually work up to a full minute. It also suggests that students work up to performing the Third through Ninth Exercises seven times each. So the complete original Mentalphysics routine is First and Second Exercises as described above, then the Third through Ninth Exercises seven times each, with each of those breaths held for a minute.

Energetic effect for Third through Ninth Mentalphysics Exercises: Squeezing the PC muscle compresses and drives prana strongly from the lower chakras to the upper chakras in all of these exercises and from there out to your arms and legs. It's so powerful that you should absolutely *not* hold your breath for any longer than five seconds. You only have to perform the First through Ninth Exercises *one time*, rather than seven times each, which is what the original exercises recommend.

The Fourth Mentalphysics Exercise: The Inspirational Breath

Starting position: Same as Revitalizing Breath.

Exercise: Exhale through the mouth. Begin your inhalation, raise your arms to the sides, and gradually swing them out and move them overhead. Keep them straight and fairly tensed throughout. Time your inhalation so that your arms are directly overhead when your inhalation is full and complete. At that highest point, the backs of your hands should be touching (Photo 12–l). Then sniff audibly and lock the breath in your body. Tense your body and squeeze the PC muscle. Hold your breath and bodily tension for five seconds. As you bring your arms down, pause for a moment at three points on the clock: arms at 2:00 and 10:00; arms at 3:00 and 9:00; arms at 4:00 and 7:00 (Photo 12–m). At each pause release a portion of your breath in a burst through your clenched teeth. As your hands come down to your sides, release the rest of your breath, then release your bodily tension. Perform one cycle of pranic breathing and then relax and be aware of your body for a few moments.

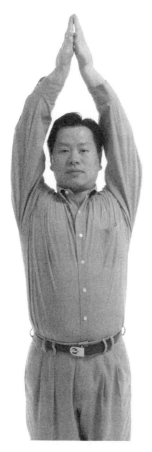

PHOTO 12–l

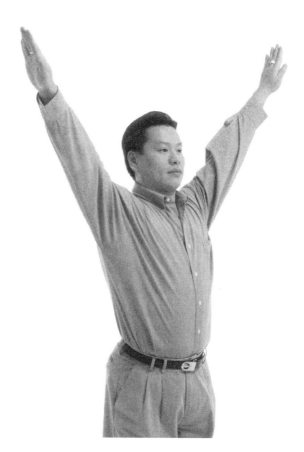

PHOTO 12–m

The Fifth Mentalphysics Exercise: The Perfection Breath

Starting position: Same as Revitalizing Breath.

Exercise: Exhale through the mouth. Begin your inhalation, raise your arms to shoulder height directly in front of you, and form your hands into fists (Photo 12–n). Keep them straight and fairly tensed throughout. Then sniff audibly, and lock the breath in your body. Tense your body, and squeeze the PC muscle. As you hold your breath and this

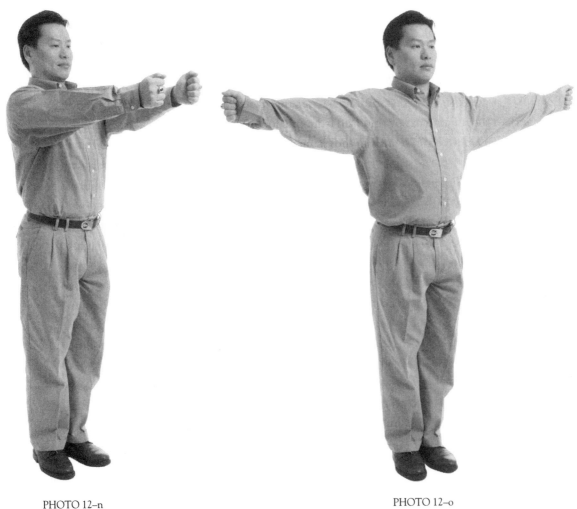

PHOTO 12–n   PHOTO 12–o

bodily tension, swing your arms directly outward to the side. At their farthest point, your arms should be outstretched and in the form of a cross (Photo 12–o). Then bring the arms back to the front. Perform this swinging motion smoothly two more times, for a total of three times. Then return to your starting position by bringing your hands down to your sides and unballing your fists. Exhale, then release your bodily tension. Perform one cycle of pranic breathing and then relax and be aware of your body for a few moments.

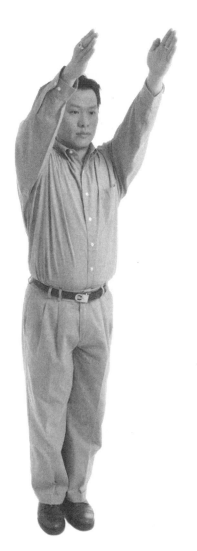

The Sixth Mentalphysics Exercise: The Vibro-Magnetic Breath

Starting position: Same as Revitalizing Breath.

Exercise: Exhale through the mouth. Inhale fully, then sniff and lock in the breath. Tense the body and squeeze the PC muscle. While holding your breath and keeping your muscles tense, swing your arms upward and forward. Swing them over your head in a backwards circular movement (Photo 12–p). Keep them straight and tensed throughout. Try to move them in a complete circle over your head and back, though the shoulder's anatomy will prevent all but the most limber or double-jointed people from making a perfect circle. This is fine. Don't dislocate your shoulder. Perform three backward rotations while holding your breath and keeping your body and PC muscle tense. Then return to your starting position by bringing your hands down to your side. Exhale, then release your bodily tension. Perform one cycle of pranic breathing and then relax and be aware of your body for a few moments.

PHOTO 12–p

The Seventh Mentalphysics Exercise: The Cleansing Breath

Starting position: Same as Revitalizing Breath. Then place your hands at your coccyx or directly over the basic chakra. Place the back of one hand against your body and the back of the other hand in the palm of the hand that is resting against the body. Your arms will bend at the elbow, but still keep them tense. This posture forces your shoulders back and your chest out (Photo 12–q).

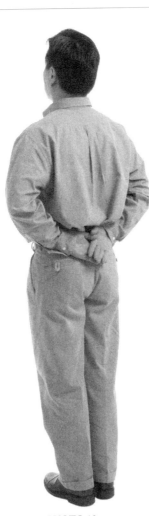

PHOTO 12–q

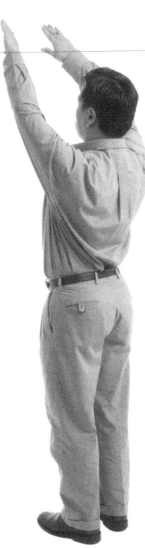

PHOTO 12–r

Exercise: Exhale through the mouth. Inhale fully, then sniff audibly and lock in the breath. Tense the body, and squeeze the PC muscle. While holding your breath and keeping your muscles tense, unlock your hands and swing your arms upward and forward. Swing them over your head in the same type of backward circular movement you used in the Vibro-Magnetic Breath (Photo 12–r). If your arms are bent and your circle isn't perfect, that's fine, but keep the arms fairly tensed throughout. Bring your hands back to the coccyx after the revolution. Perform two more of these rotations for a total of three. Bring your hands back to the coccyx after each revolution. Then return to your original starting position by bringing your hands down to your sides. Exhale, then release your bodily tension. Perform one cycle of pranic breathing and then relax and be aware of your body for a few moments.

Key modification for Seventh Mentalphysics Exercise: The original Mentalphysics program calls for you to lock your arms behind your back and keep them straight, which places strain on the shoulders. This modification makes it easier to perform the exercise.

The Eighth Mentalphysics Exercise: The Grand Rejuvenation Breath

Starting position: Same as Revitalizing Breath. Then place your hands on your hips with your thumbs resting on your hip bones and the fingers moving forward into your abdominal area. Move your elbows forward so that your back fans out (Photo 12–s).

Exercise: Exhale through the mouth. Inhale fully, then sniff and lock in the breath. Tense the body, and squeeze the PC muscle. While holding your breath and keeping your muscles tense, pivot your head forward until your chin is resting on your chest; then move it back as far as it will comfortably go. Perform this back-and-forth movement three times smoothly while holding your breath. Bring your head back to the starting position and exhale fully. Then, *without inhaling* and while keeping your body—and especially your legs and buttocks—tense, pivot forward on your hips until your upper body is perpendicular to the floor (or as far forward as is comfortable for you), then bend backward as far as you can comfortably go. Perform this back-and-forth movement three times smoothly (Photo 12–t). Then return to your starting position by bringing your hands down to your sides, and release your bodily tension. Perform one cycle of pranic breathing and then relax and be aware of your body for a few moments.

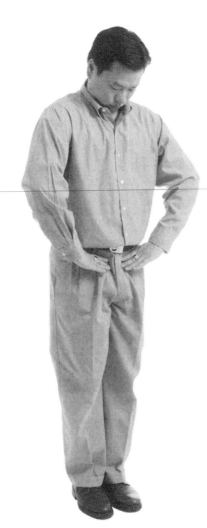

PHOTO 12–s

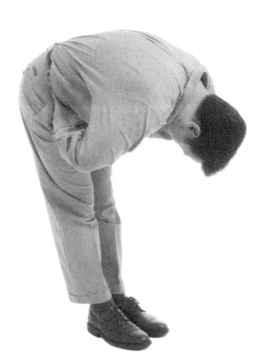

PHOTO 12–t

The Ninth Mentalphysics Exercise: The Spiritual Breath

Starting position: Same as the Grand Rejuvenation Breath, except that your feet are shoulder-width apart (Photo 12–u).

Exercise: Exhale through the mouth. Inhale fully, then sniff and lock in the breath. Tense the body, and squeeze the PC muscle. While holding your breath and keeping your muscles tense, bend or lean straight over to the right as far as you comfortably can, until your left heel lifts off the ground (Photo 12–v). Then reverse the movement and bend

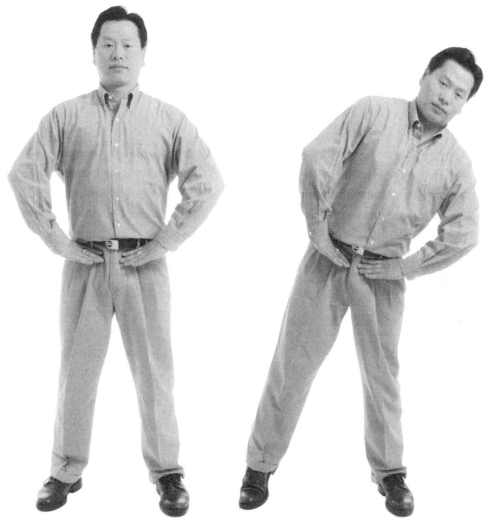

PHOTO 12–u   PHOTO 12–v

241

or lean straight over to the left, until your right heel lifts off the ground. Perform this movement for a total of three times in each direction. Then return to your starting position by bringing your hands down to your sides. Exhale, then release your bodily tension. Perform one cycle of pranic breathing and then relax and be aware of your body for a few moments.

After you complete the exercises, simply walk around and stretch a bit and resume your daily activities.

SIX STEPS DAILY PRACTICE ROUTINE—UPDATE

The optimum time to practice the Tibetan Yogic Exercises or Mentalphysics Exercises is immediately after you meditate. Here is a good sequence for incorporating energy-generating exercises into your daily routine:

1. Invoke for guidance and protection.
2. Cut cords.
3. Do cleansing physical exercises.
4. Do pranic breathing.
5. Do direct clearing techniques, as needed.
6. Meditate (alternate Mindfulness with Twin Hearts, according to your schedule and preference).
7. Do cleansing physical exercises after meditation.
8. Do energy-generating exercises (either Tibetan Yogic Exercises or Mentalphysics Exercises; after attaining proficiency, you can alternate them daily as well).
9. Do the standard warm-up.
10. Do hand sensitivity, scanning, sweeping, energizing practice.
11. Do special exercises: general self-sweeping, general stress-relief, work/house cleaning, and so on.

Add energetic hygiene practices as needed, or as you have time.

You now have learned all six steps to self-healing. In the next chapter, in Part III, you will learn energetic remedies for 24 common health problems.

Part III

Staying Energized and Healthy

CHAPTER 13

A Self-Healing Guide—
Energetic Solutions
to 24 Common
Health Problems

"I have used Pranic Healing to relieve headaches, restore emotional stability and calmness, overcome constipation, anesthetize insect bites, and soothe skin rashes. For example, to relieve constipation, I sweep the ascending, transverse, and descending colon, alternating with light whitish-green and light whitish-orange; I do the same for the base of the spine. To relieve headaches, I sweep the ajna *counterclockwise with light whitish-green and light whitish-violet, and solar plexus front and back with light whitish-green and light whitish-orange."*

—Kenneth Klee, Los Angeles

This chapter is the culmination of your energy-manipulation work. It contains scanning, sweeping, and energizing remedies for 24 common health ailments, plus a special pre- and postsurgery energetic routine. You might think of this chapter as a self-healing "cookbook," with each remedy a "recipe." For each problem, follow the step-by-step instructions for sweeping and energizing the indicated area(s) and chakra(s) with the indicated color(s). Each sequence has been designed to address the specific remedy indicated. Although we encourage students to try creative applications of their self-healing work, it's probably best that you follow the instructions in this chapter closely in the beginning. You can experiment after you become a more proficient healer.

ENERGY HEALING SUCCESS FACTORS

At the outset of your energy healing work, it's appropriate to recap the energy healing success factors, in their order of importance:

1. *Intent*. Establishing a clear intent—to scan, to sweep, or to increase and project prana—is the most important factor in successful energy healing work. Clear, firm, sincere intent overcomes lack of experience and even the inability to feel the energy and visualize.

2. *Technique*. While you needn't tie yourself into knots trying to put your fingers in the exact same angles that you see in the illustrations in this book, you do need a certain amount of precision in your hand postures and movements in energy healing. Some elements of certain techniques are more critical than others. For example, the hand movement in local sweeping is *always* counterclockwise. If you clean with a clockwise motion, you're using the movement for energizing, and that may aggravate the condition. You should also adhere closely to the step-by-step energetic remedies in this chapter; they are proven, tested sequences. The visualization technique that is "best" for you, though, is a matter of individual preference; use the one that works most effectively for you. We've indicated throughout where you can deviate from the recommended routine and how much latitude is acceptable.

3. *Ability to sense or feel prana*. It is undoubtedly helpful to be able to feel the energy, but it is not essential that you have a strong sensitivity to energy for the remedies to work. Some people take longer than two weeks to get the requisite sensitivity, yet they can still get the benefit of the healing routines if their intent is clear and strong. And as noted many times, you can still perform healings if you can't feel the energy.

4. *Ability to visualize clearly*. Clear, crisp pictures of your healing are also helpful, particularly if you're a visual person. But your visualization of, for instance, the back of the body as you sweep and energize the back chakras doesn't have to be perfect. Some people simply have a difficult time imagining and maintaining pictures, yet they are still effective self-healers. Again, if your intent is firm, it can compensate for less-than-photo-quality visualizations.

To sum up the energy healing success factors, it is *essential* to have clear intent, it is *important* to have proper technique, it is *good* to be able to feel the prana, and it's *helpful* to be able to visualize well.

PROBLEMS ASSOCIATED WITH SELF-HEALING AND SOME SOLUTIONS

There are two principal roadblocks that people encounter in self-healing: first, weakness, pain, or fatigue that make concentration or focus difficult; and second, an understandable tendency to focus on the problem rather than on the remedy. If you have the flu, often all you want to do is sit around and watch television. Or if you have a headache, you just want to go into a dark room and lie down. If you're tired or in pain, it may be a challenge to gear yourself up for self-healing. Additionally, when you're feeling physically down, you may also be mentally down; it may be difficult *not* to think about your aching head, your queasy stomach, or your swollen knee.

Here are a couple of tips to deal with these problems:

1. *Practice good energetic hygiene.* Take a salt bath, eat energetically clean foods, and take cleansing and energizing herbs or supplements to kick-start your energy when you're tired. Good energetic hygiene builds up your strength and also gives your willpower a boost. This enables you to take more forceful self-healing steps.

2. *Acknowledge your situation.* As you've read, it's not productive to deny or suppress your negative emotions. It's the same with your physical condition. If you have an extremely sore back, telling yourself over and over "My back is fine" isn't positive mental attitude or reinforcement. It's self-delusion and actually self-defeating because your unconscious mind knows your back isn't right. You can't ignore your current health circumstances. Be clear-eyed about your situation. If you're weak, hurting, or tired, acknowledge it but don't focus on it or be obsessed with it. Be objective.

3. *Perform pranic breathing and cleansing physical exercises.* This will build up your willpower and strength.

4. *Sweep and energize your* ajna. This will also build up your will. Sweep your *ajna* 50 times (10 sets of five counterclockwise sweeps, alternating green and violet) and then energize it with white prana for 10 cycles of pranic breathing. This reinforces your resolve to take further self-healing action.

5. *Finally, don't hesitate to seek out traditional medical advice.* We advocate a complementary approach to healing that includes both traditional and alternative methods. Many traditional remedies have a basis in energetic truth—for example, highly sensitive healers who can see energy in its various colors note that ibuprofen is filled with luminous blue-green prana, which is the optimal color prana for reducing inflammation. For some

problems, you may need a procedure or a prescription to supplement your own self-healing. So don't hesitate to seek the advice of a physician or traditional health care practitioner if necessary.

A Few Final Notes on Energetic Remedies Before You Begin

- You will see that the colors in the remedies are now described as "light whitish-green," or "light whitish-blue" instead of "light green " or "light blue" or even "green" or "blue." These terms don't change how you use or visualize colors. They merely help remind you to keep the colors pastel, not dark. When you energize with light whitish-green, you still use a bright white disk with a pastel ring of pale green around it. When you sweep with light whitish-violet, you still use a very pale beam of violet.

- "Sweeping," unless otherwise specified, always refers to "local sweeping," which means you'd use either the dog paddle or the counterclockwise motion.

- "Stabilize" means to paint an area you just worked on with light blue to keep the prana in place.

- "Inhibit" means to energize with light whitish-blue or sometimes with a darker shade of blue with intent to *reduce* the size and energy of a chakra.

- "Sweeping alternately" with colors means to sweep with two sets of five sweeps with one color (e.g., light whitish-green), then with two sets of five sweeps of another color (e.g., light whitish-violet). Continue alternating the colors like that as you sweep. Spray your hands with alcohol after every ten total sweeps.

- A few remedies include work on several minor chakras that haven't been mentioned up to this point. You sweep and energize them as directed, just as you do with the major chakras. The location of each minor chakra is indicated.

- Energy healing can produce amazing—and often immediate—results. In the beginning of your practice, however, the healing effects may not come as quickly as you might expect. Remember that there can be a lag time, and as you build up proficiency and the ability to draw in more prana, this lag time will be diminished.

- If you are uncomfortable with using colors, or don't feel confident in your ability to project colors, you can simply follow the remedies using white rather than colored prana for both sweeping and energizing.

- As noted earlier, if you are working on a woman who is pregnant or who you suspect may be pregnant, you should perform only sweeping and only with white prana.

- Many factors affect healing: aptitude for energy manipulation, the seriousness of the ailment, and how long it has persisted, to name just a few. So it's difficult to give one standard recommendation for how long to sweep and energize and how frequently to apply each remedy. It's best to use the general guidelines you've already learned. So unless otherwise indicated in the remedy:

Use at least an 80 to 20 percent sweeping-to-energizing ratio.

Sweep in passes or counterclockwise revolutions in sets of ten (actually, two sets of five).

Energize for five to seven cycles of pranic breathing for simple problems and 10 or more for complex or long-lasting problems.

Here's how it works in the remedy for migraine. The first step is to work on the front solar plexus chakra. Since most migraines are complex problems, you would energize with each color for 10 cycles of pranic breathing. To maintain the 80:20 sweeping-to-energizing ratio, you would precede your energizing by sweeping with each color for 40 counterclockwise revolutions of your hand.

Thus in the first step you sweep the front solar plexus chakra with light whitish-green 40 times, then light whitish-blue 40 times, then light whitish-violet 40 times in sets of five (spraying with alcohol after each ten sweeps). After you are completely finished sweeping, you then energize with light whitish-green for 10 cycles of pranic breathing, then with light whitish-blue for 10 cycles of pranic breathing, then with light whitish-violet for 10 cycles of pranic breathing. Then stabilize, inhibit, and move on to the next step in the sequence until you complete all the steps.

Unless otherwise indicated, perform the remedy once daily until the problem improves or goes away. Use your own judgment and scanning ability, as well. If you are feeling better and scanning reveals that the energy level in the affected area(s) is normal, you're done.

(*Note:* While these are extremely effective, powerful energetic remedies for the problems listed, we regard them as complementary techniques, to be used along with traditional medicine, and any other preventive, dietary, holistic, or alternative treatments you've found to be helpful for your particular condition.)

1. ARTHRITIS, JOINT INFLAMMATION

1. Affected joint or area: Sweep alternately with light whitish-green and light whitish-blue for at least 5 minutes. Energize with light whitish-green, then light whitish-blue, then light whitish-violet. Stabilize. These two steps provide immediate but temporary relief. For more long-lasting relief, add the following two steps.

2. Front solar plexus chakra: Sweep with light whitish-green, then energize with white prana. Stabilize.

3. Repeat step 2 on the back solar plexus, sex, navel, and basic chakras. Energize the basic with light whitish-red to strengthen the musculoskeletal system.

2. ASTHMA

1. General sweeping with light whitish-green.
2. Throat chakra: Sweep with light whitish-green, then energize with light whitish-green, then light whitish-red. Red prana has a dilating effect on the air passageway. Stabilize.
3. Lungs: Sweep with light whitish-green, then light whitish-orange. Energize the lungs directly through the back with light whitish-green, then light whitish-orange, then light whitish-red. When energizing the lungs with orange prana, your fingers should be pointed outward and away from the head. If you are unsure of your control or color, simply omit light whitish-orange. Stabilize. Orange prana has an expelling effect, which enhances the dilating and strengthening effects of the red prana.
4. Front solar plexus chakra: Sweep with light whitish-green, then energize with light whitish-green, then light whitish-violet. Stabilize.
5. Repeat step 4 on the back solar plexus chakra and the liver.
6. If the asthma is stress- or emotion-related, activate the heart chakra in this way: Sweep the front heart chakra with light whitish-green. Then sweep the back heart chakra with light whitish-green and energize the heart chakra through the back heart chakra with light whitish-green, then light whitish-violet. Stabilize. This sequence regulates the lower emotions and produces a sense of inner peace.
7. Basic chakra: Sweep with light whitish-green, then energize with light whitish-red. Stabilize.
8. *Ajna* chakra: Sweep alternately with light whitish-green and light whitish-violet. Energize with light whitish-green, then light whitish-violet. Stabilize.
9. Repeat three times a week. For preventive healing, you can also apply the technique whenever you feel the slightest sensation of shortness of breath.

3. BACKACHE

1. General sweeping with light whitish-green.
2. Entire spine: Sweep with light whitish-green seven times.
3. Front solar plexus chakra: Sweep with light whitish-green. Energize with light whitish-green, then light whitish-blue, then light whitish-violet. Stabilize.
4. Repeat the above sequence for the back solar plexus chakra and the liver.

5. Front heart chakra: Sweep with light whitish-green.

6. Back heart chakra: Sweep with light whitish-green. Energize the back heart chakra with light whitish-green, then light whitish-violet. Simultaneously visualize the heart chakra becoming bigger.

7. Affected area: Sweep alternately with light whitish-green and light whitish-orange. Energize with light whitish-green, then light whitish-blue, then light whitish-yellow. Stabilize.

8. Basic chakra: Sweep with light whitish-green, then energize with light whitish-red. Stabilize.

4. BLADDER WEAKNESS, URINARY URGENCY AND FREQUENCY, URINARY TRACT INFECTION

1. General sweeping two times with light whitish-green.

2. Sex chakra: Sweep alternately with light whitish-green and light whitish-orange. Energize with light whitish-green, then light whitish-blue, then light whitish-violet.

3. Surrounding lower abdominal area: Sweep alternately with light whitish-green and light whitish-orange.

4. Sex chakra: Energize again with light whitish-green, then light whitish-blue, then light whitish-violet. Stabilize.

5. Lungs, front and back: Sweep alternately with light whitish-green and light whitish-orange, then energize through the back with light whitish-green, then light whitish-orange. This facilitates healing since it has a cleansing effect on the blood and the entire body. When energizing the lungs with orange prana, your fingers should be pointed outward and away from the head. If you are unsure of your control or color, simply omit light whitish-orange.

6. Front solar plexus chakra: Sweep with light whitish-green, then energize with white. Stabilize.

7. Repeat step 6 on the back solar plexus, navel, and basic chakras. This sequence strengthens the body and enhances the body's immunity and defense system.

8. These ailments respond particularly well to treatment, but they consume prana rapidly. Thus, repeat treatment two to three times a day, if possible, for several days.

5. BURNS

1. Affected area: Sweep alternately with light whitish-green and light whitish-blue. Energize with light greenish-blue, then light whitish-violet. Stabilize.

2. Basic chakra: Sweep with light whitish-green, then energize with light whitish-red. Stabilize.

6. CARPAL TUNNEL / REPETITIVE MOTION INJURIES OF THE HAND OR ARM

1. Affected joint or area: Sweep alternately with light whitish-green and light whitish-blue for at least 5 minutes. Energize with whitish-green, then light whitish-blue, then light whitish-violet. Stabilize.
2. Repeat step 1 on the armpit, jaw, and back of the head.
3. Front solar plexus chakra: Sweep with light whitish-green, then energize with white prana. Stabilize.
4. Repeat step 2 on the back solar plexus, navel, and basic chakras.

7. COLD, INFLUENZA, SINUSITIS, LUNG INFECTION, BRONCHITIS, PNEUMONIA, FEVER

1. General sweeping two times with light whitish-green.
2. Front solar plexus chakra: Sweep alternately with light whitish-green and light whitish-violet, then energize with light whitish-green and then light whitish-blue. Stabilize.
3. Repeat step 2 on the back solar plexus chakra.
4. Liver: Sweep with light whitish-green.
5. Front heart chakra: Sweep with light whitish-green.
6. Back heart chakra: Sweep with light whitish-green, then energize with light whitish-green, then light whitish-violet. Stabilize. Sweep again with light whitish-green.
7. Lungs: Sweep with light whitish-green. Energize the lungs directly but carefully through the back with light whitish-green, light whitish-orange, and then light whitish-violet. When energizing the lungs with orange prana, your fingers should be pointed outward and away from the head. If you are unsure of your control or color, simply omit light whitish-orange.
8. *Ajna* chakra: Sweep with light whitish-green. Energize with light whitish-green, then light whitish-blue, then light whitish-violet. Stabilize.
9. Repeat step 8 on the throat chakra.
10. Front spleen chakra: Sweep with light-whitish green, then gently energize with white prana. Stabilize.
11. Repeat step 10 on the back spleen chakra.

12. Navel chakra: Sweep with light whitish-green, then energize with white prana. Stabilize.
13. Repeat step 12 on the basic chakra.
14. Arms and legs: Sweep with light whitish-green, then energize with light whitish-violet.
15. Repeat step 14 on the palm chakras (the chakras used in hand sensitivity and scanning). Work on the left with the right and vice versa.
16. Repeat at least once a day until the problem is resolved. It is especially helpful to perform the technique as soon as any symptoms appear.

8. CONSTIPATION

1. Front solar plexus chakra: Sweep with light whitish-green, then energize with light whitish-green, then light whitish-red. Sweep again with light whitish-green.
2. Repeat step 1 on the back solar plexus chakra.
3. Navel chakra: Sweep with light whitish-green, then energize with light whitish-green, light whitish-orange, then light whitish-red. Sweep again alternately with light whitish-green and light whitish-orange. (Green cleanses, orange eliminates, red strengthens.)
4. Sweep entire abdominal area with light whitish-green.
5. Basic chakra: Sweep with whitish-green, then energize with light whitish-red prana. Stabilize.

9. DEPRESSION (MILD)

1. Cord-cutting: Visualize out in front of you the incident or cause of the negative thoughts or emotions, then sever the cord from it at the solar plexus area. Then visualize throwing it into a violet fire.
2. General sweeping seven times with light whitish-green, then seven times with electric violet.
3. Front solar plexus chakra: Form a clear intent that you are sweeping away any negative thoughts and emotions lodged in that chakra. Then sweep with electric violet for up to 5 minutes. Energize with electric violet for up to 5 minutes. Stabilize.
4. Repeat step 3 on the back solar plexus, throat, *ajna*, and crown chakras.
5. Navel chakra: Sweep with light whitish-green, then energize with light whitish-red. Stabilize.
6. Repeat step 5 on the basic chakra.

7. Hand (palm) and sole minor chakras: (Hand chakras are the same ones used in hand sensitivity and scanning. Sole minor chakras are located between the ball of the foot and the arch.) Sweep with light whitish-green. Energize each area with light whitish-red. Do not stabilize the palms or the soles of the feet.

10. DIET AND APPETITE CONTROL

1. Cord-cutting: Visualize out in front of you the food that you want to abstain from, then sever the cord from it at the solar plexus area. Then visualize throwing the food into a violet fire.
2. Front solar plexus chakra: Form a firm intent that with every sweep, you are removing any thoughts about, cravings for, and emotional attachments to food. Then sweep alternately with light whitish-green and electric violet. Energize with electric violet and then medium whitish-blue to inhibit the size of the chakra.
3. Throat chakra: Form a firm intent that with every sweep, you are removing any thoughts about, cravings for, and emotional attachments to food. Then sweep alternately with light whitish-green and electric violet. Energize with electric violet. Stabilize.
4. Repeat step 3 on the *ajna* chakra.
5. (Optional) Practice Meditation on Twin Hearts to accelerate the purging of negative thoughts and emotions related to food cravings.

11. EARACHE

1. Ear minor chakras (located at the ear hole): Sweep alternately with light whitish-green and light whitish-violet. Energize with light whitish-green, then light whitish-blue, then light whitish-violet. Stabilize.
2. Repeat step 1 on the jaw minor chakras and the back of the head. (The jaw minor chakra is located directly below the earlobe, at the 90-degree angle of the jawbone.)

12. EYESTRAIN

1. *Ajna* chakra: Sweep alternately with light whitish-green and light whitish-violet.
2. Energize with light whitish-green, then light whitish-blue, then light whitish-violet. Stabilize.
3. Repeat step 1 on the temples and back of the head.
4. Eyes: Sweep with light whitish-green, but do not energize.

13. FOOD POISONING, VOMITING OR DIARRHEA

1. Front solar plexus chakras: Sweep with light whitish-green. Energize with light whitish-green, then light whitish-blue, then light whitish-violet. Stabilize. Sweep again with light whitish-green.

2. Repeat step 1 on the back solar plexus and navel chakras.

3. Lower abdominal area: Sweep with light whitish-green.

4. One or two treatments is usually enough, but repeat as necessary.

14. HYPERTENSION

1. General sweeping two or three times with light whitish-green and then once with light whitish-blue.

2. Entire head area—especially the back part—plus the spine: Sweep alternately with light whitish-green and light whitish-blue.

3. Front solar plexus and back solar plexus chakras: Sweep alternately with light whitish-green and light whitish-blue. Stabilize. Inhibit.

4. *Meng mein* chakra: Sweep alternately with light whitish-green and light whitish-blue. Stabilize. Inhibit.

5. For immediate help, repeat steps 2 through 4 every two hours.

6. Front heart chakra: Sweep with light whitish-green.

7. Back heart chakra: Sweep with light whitish-green. Energize the back heart chakra with light whitish-green, then light whitish-violet. Simultaneously visualize the heart chakra becoming bigger. This sequence helps normalize blood pressure.

8. Head area: Sweep again with light whitish-green and light whitish-violet.

9. Crown chakra: Lightly energize with light whitish-green, then light whitish-blue, then light whitish-violet. Green is for cleansing, blue is for pliability of the blood vessels in the head, and violet is for strengthening. Stabilize. *Do not overenergize the head.*

10.. Repeat step 9 on the forehead and *ajna* chakras. Rescan the head and sweep again.

11. Throat chakra: Sweep with light whitish-green, then energize lightly with some light whitish-green, then more light whitish-violet. Stabilize.

12. Basic chakra: Sweep with light whitish-green, then energize slightly with light whitish-blue. Stabilize.

13. Repeat treatment several times a week if necessary.

15. INSOMNIA

1. Cord-cutting: Visualize out in front of you any incident or cause of any negative

thoughts or emotions that could be bothering you, then sever the cord from it at the solar plexus area. Then visualize throwing it into a violet fire.

2. General sweeping two times with light whitish-green.

3. Front solar plexus chakra: Sweep with light whitish-green, then light whitish-blue. Stabilize. Inhibit.

4. Repeat step 3 on the back solar plexus, *meng mein*, and basic chakras.

5. Crown chakra: Sweep with light whitish-green.

6. Repeat step 5 on the forehead, *ajna*, and throat chakras.

7. Navel chakra: Sweep with light whitish-green, then energize with white prana. Stabilize.

8. Sweep the whole spine downward with the intent to sweep away any excess, negative, or dirty energy that is flowing up to the head and neck areas.

16. IRRITABLE BOWEL SYNDROME

1. Front solar plexus chakra: Sweep with light whitish-green. Energize with light whitish-green, then light whitish-blue, then light whitish-violet. Stabilize.

2. Repeat step 1 on the back solar plexus and navel chakras.

17. MENSTRUAL CRAMPS AND DISCOMFORT

1. General sweeping seven times with light whitish-green.

2. Sex chakra: Sweep alternately with light whitish-green and light whitish-orange. Energize with light whitish-green, then light whitish-orange, then light whitish-red. Stabilize.

3. Navel chakra: Sweep with light whitish-green, then energize with white prana. Stabilize.

4. Repeat step 3 on the basic chakra.

5. For best results, perform the techniques once a day beginning three days prior to the menstrual period. Continue during the period as well.

18. MIGRAINE HEADACHE

1. Front solar plexus chakra: Sweep with light whitish-green, then light whitish-blue, then light whitish-violet. Energize with light whitish-green, then light whitish-blue, then light whitish-violet. Stabilize. Inhibit.

2. Repeat the above sequence for the back solar plexus and *meng mein* chakras.

3. Liver: Sweep with light whitish-green, then light whitish-blue.

4. Spine and upper back: Sweep with light whitish-green, then light whitish-blue. Sweep downward with the intent to sweep away any negative or dirty energy that is flowing up to the head and neck areas.

5. Front heart chakra: Sweep with light whitish-green.

6. Back heart chakra: Sweep with light whitish-green. Energize the back heart chakra lightly with light whitish-green, then light whitish-violet. Visualize the heart chakra becoming bigger.

7. (*Note:* For steps 7 and 8, use a ratio of 9:1 sweeping-to-energizing ratio.) Affected head area(s): Sweep with light whitish-green, then light whitish-blue. Energize with light whitish-green, then light whitish-blue, then light whitish-violet. Stabilize.

8. Repeat step 7 on the *ajna*, forehead, and crown chakras.

19. NEGATIVE THOUGHTS (PERSISTENT)

1. Cord-cutting: Visualize out in front of you the incident or the cause of the negative thoughts or emotions, then sever the cord from it at the solar plexus area. Then visualize throwing it into a violet fire.

2. Front solar plexus chakra: Form a firm intent that any negative thoughts and emotions be completely removed. Then sweep with electric violet for at least 5 minutes.

3. Energize with electric violet for about 2 minutes. Stabilize. Inhibit.

4. Repeat step 2 on the back solar plexus, throat, *ajna*, and crown chakras.

5. (Optional) Perform Meditation on Twin Hearts to rapidly flush out negative thoughts and emotions from the entire aura.

20. PAIN RELIEF (GENERAL), PRANIC ANESTHESIA

(*Note:* Pranic anesthesia is used before a procedure only, e.g., dental work. Don't use it to numb an injury that needs to be repaired. Use another remedy instead, perhaps the ones for sprains/athletic injuries or arthritis/joint inflammation.)

1. Affected area: Energize with light whitish-greenish-blue for two to three cycles of pranic breathing. Visualize the energy filling up the area.

2. Energize with medium blue for two to three cycles of pranic breathing. (*Note:* This is one of the very few times you'll use a darker color.)

3. Energize with light whitish-violet for one cycle of pranic breathing.

4. Stabilize.

21. SORE THROAT

1. Entire throat area: Sweep alternately with light whitish-green and light whitish-violet. Energize with light whitish-green, then light whitish-blue, then light whitish-violet. Stabilize.
2. Repeat step 1 on the jaw minor chakras and throat chakra.
3. Repeat steps 1 and 2 until you experience relief.

22. SPRAINS AND SPORTS INJURIES TO JOINTS AND MUSCLES

1. Affected area: Sweep alternately with light whitish-green and light whitish-orange. Energize with light whitish-blue (for pain relief, soothing, and stabilizing). Energize with light whitish-orange, then light whitish-red, then light whitish-yellow. Repeat until there is substantial relief.
2. Basic chakra: Sweep with light whitish-green, then energize with light whitish-red. Stabilize.
3. Repeat step 2 on the navel chakra.
4. Don't overexert the area immediately.

23. STRESS RELIEF (GENERAL)

(*Note:* There are a number of ways to relieve stress. This remedy is similar to—but more comprehensive, more thorough, and longer than—the one you learned in Chapter 9. Exercise 9-F can be used for lighter episodes of stress or when you have less time. Experiment and see which works better for you.)

1. Cord-cutting: Visualize out in front of you the incident or stimulus of the negative thoughts or emotions, then sever the cord from it at the solar plexus area. Then visualize throwing it into a violet fire.
2. General sweeping seven times with light whitish-green, then seven times with electric violet.
3. Front and back solar plexus chakras: Form a clear intent to sweep away any negative thoughts and emotions lodged in the chakras, then sweep with electric violet for up to 5 minutes. Energize with electric violet for up to 5 minutes. Stabilize. Inhibit.
4. Repeat step 3 on the *ajna*, throat, and crown chakras, but do not inhibit.
5. (Optional) Perform Meditation on Twin Hearts to rapidly flush out negative thoughts and emotions from the entire aura.

24. ULCER

1. Stomach and small intestines: Sweep alternately with light whitish-green and light whitish-violet.
2. Front solar plexus chakra: Sweep alternately with light whitish-green and light whitish-violet, then energize with light whitish-blue, then light whitish-violet.
3. Repeat step 2 on the back solar plexus and navel chakras.
4. Sweep and energize alternately on all these areas until you experience relief.
5. Front heart chakra: Sweep with light whitish-green, then light whitish-violet.
6. Repeat step 5 on the back heart chakra. Then energize the heart chakra through the back heart chakra with light whitish-green prana, then light whitish-violet. Stabilize. This sequence activates the heart chakra and produces a sense of inner peace.
7. Basic chakra: Sweep with light whitish-green, then energize with light whitish-red. Stabilize.
8. Repeat treatment two to three times a week.

SPECIAL PRE- AND POST-SURGERY ROUTINES

These special advanced routines can be used on anyone who undergoes surgery. The pre-surgery routine strengthens the aura and enables it to withstand the rapid escape of prana from the body after an incision is made. It should be performed *for at least three consecutive days prior to the day of surgery.* The post-surgery routine removes the dirty, grayish energy that surrounds and clogs the entire body after surgery and helps accelerate the body's ability to repair itself. It should be performed daily *for at least four days after surgery.*

Pre-surgery:

1. General sweeping alternately with light whitish-green and light whitish-violet, 10 times each color.
2. Sweep and straighten the health rays.
3. Area to be operated on: Sweep alternately with light whitish-green and light whitish violet, 10 times each color. Energize with light whitish-green, then light whitish-violet, for at least 5 minutes. Stabilize.
4. Basic chakra: Sweep alternately with light whitish-green and light whitish-violet, 10 times each color. Energize with light whitish-red for at least 5 minutes. Stabilize.
5. Repeat step 4 on the navel chakra.

6. Front and back solar plexus chakras: Sweep alternately with light whitish-green and light whitish violet, 10 times each color. Energize with white prana for at least 5 minutes. Stabilize.

Post-surgery:

1. General sweeping alternately with light whitish-green and light whitish-violet, 30 times each color. You will find that the aura is usually very murky, heavy, and dirty.
2. Sweep and straighten the health rays.
3. Area operated on: Sweep alternately with light whitish-green and light whitish-violet, 50 times each color. Energize with light whitish-green, then light whitish-violet, for at least 10 minutes each color, alternating colors every 2 minutes. Stabilize.
4. Basic chakra: Sweep alternately with light whitish-green and light whitish-violet, 50 times each color. Energize with light whitish-red for at least 10 minutes. Stabilize.
5. Repeat step 4 on the navel chakra.
6. Front and back solar plexus chakras: Sweep alternately with light whitish-green and light whitish-violet, 100 times each color. Energize with white prana for at least 10 minutes. Stabilize.

SIX STEPS DAILY PRACTICE ROUTINE—UPDATE

Self-healing routines can be practiced alone, as needed, or in the context of a daily routine. If you include them as part of a full daily routine, the optimal point in your sequence to perform them is after meditation or during the "special exercises" section. See below.

1. Invoke for guidance and protection.
2. Cut cords.
3. Do cleansing physical exercises.
4. Do pranic breathing.
5. Do direct clearing techniques, as needed.
6. Meditate (alternate Mindfulness with Twin Hearts, according to your schedule and preference).
7. Cleansing physical exercises after meditation.
   (*Add self-healings.*)

8. Do energy-generating exercises (initially, pick either Tibetan Yogic Exercises or Mentalphysics Exercises; after attaining proficiency, can alternate them daily as well).
9. Do the standard warm-up.
10. Do hand sensitivity, scanning, sweeping, energizing practice.
11. Do special exercises: general self-sweeping, general stress-reduction, work/house cleaning. (*Add self-healings.*)

Add energetic hygiene techniques as needed, or as you have time available.

In the next chapter, you'll learn to pull together all your work to this point into a regular energy-boosting health maintenance routine.

CHAPTER 14

Prescription for Greater Energy and Better Health— The *Your Hands Can Heal You* Daily Routine

"The same day I completed my very first Pranic Healing workshop, my sister suffered a mild heart attack. As I drove to the hospital the next day, I wondered if these techniques I'd learned could help her in any way. When I arrived at the intensive care unit, the monitor registering her vital signs indicated that her blood pressure was still high despite the medications she'd been given to control it. I asked her if she would be open to this new 'thing' I had just discovered. After a short invocation for guidance, I began doing the simple techniques I had learned over the weekend: scanning, sweeping, and energizing.

"When I was done, her boyfriend stared at the monitor, his mouth open in disbelief. Her blood pressure had dropped dramatically. Still not sure if Pranic Healing had anything to do with this change, I chalked it up to the fact that she was comforted by my presence and relaxed by the swirling hand movements above her body.

"The next day she underwent a procedure to clear a blocked artery. After the procedure, I visited her, and right away she asked, 'Can you do your "thing" again?' I said I would. I noticed that her recent procedure had now left her with very low blood pressure. All I knew how to do was the basic Pranic Healing technique I had done the day before, and I was worried because I didn't want her blood pressure to drop any lower. After another invocation for guidance, I once again started my work.

"After about 45 minutes, I glanced at the monitor and was shocked! Her blood pressure was actually rising! I later realized that the Pranic Healing techniques simply allowed her body to heal itself and normalize her blood pressure in both instances. I also realized that anyone, with minimal training, can facilitate healing in themselves and others."

—MICHAEL MARTIN, RIVERSIDE, CALIFORNIA

262

This brief chapter offers a regular routine to keep you in a state of optimum health and keep your personal supply of energy consistently high. It's the culmination of all your practice routines. Include these steps in your life to the degree that you have time and to the extent that you feel comfortable. Even minimal practice has a positive effect on your health, but obviously the more regularly and diligently you practice, the better.

The morning is the best time of the day for energy work. The prana is fresher, and you're fresher energetically. Additionally, energy work is a good way to start your day. Thus, if you have only one time of the day for breathing, meditating, and self-healing, it should be the morning. Of course, if you have a schedule that makes it difficult for you to practice in the morning, of if you're not a "morning person," the routine still works any time you practice it. But we recommend that you try to do your energy work in the morning.

Consider the basic routine the baseline or minimum you should do. The moderate routine is for those who have more time. The full routine is for those who are interested in optimal results.

Morning Routine

Basic	Moderate	Full
• Invocation • Cord-cutting • Cleansing physical exercises • Pranic breathing • Meditation (three to five times per week, alternate Mindfulness and Twin Hearts) *"Basic" basic:* For mornings when you are pressed for time, you can cut cords and do the exercises and some pranic breathing; you'll still get a very good start on your day.	• Invocation • Cord-cutting • Cleansing physical exercises • Pranic breathing • Meditation (five times per week, alternating Mindfulness and Twin Hearts) • Energy-generating exercises (three to five times per week, either Tibetan Yogic Exercises or Mentalphysics Exercises; after you master them both, you can alternate them daily)	• Invocation • Cord-cutting • Cleansing physical exercises • Pranic breathing • Self-sweeping, using method of your choosing • Meditation (every day, alternating Mindfulness and Twin Hearts every other day) • Energy-generating exercises (every day, either Tibetan Yogic Exercises or Mentalphysics Exercises)

Afternoon Routine

- Midday energy boost: three sets of ten pranic breaths, followed by the first two Mental-physics breathing exercises (Balancing Breathing and Rapid Turtle Breathing)
- Specific remedies, as needed
- Cut cords, as needed

Evening Routine

Basic	Moderate	Full
• Invoke • Cut cords • Salt bath (two times per week, or as needed, depending upon level of contamination)	• Invoke • Cut cords • Salt bath (two to three times per week, or as needed, depending upon level of contamination) • Pranic breathing	• Invoke • Cut cords • Salt bath (two to three times per week, or as needed, depending upon level of contamination) • Pranic breathing • Meditation: the meditation you didn't do in your morning session

Practice or apply as needed:

- Hand sensitivity
- Scanning, sweeping, energizing practice
- Direct clearing techniques
- Special techniques (for example, work/house cleansing, closing and strengthening aura)
- Specific healing remedies
- Dietary recommendations
- Physical exercise

In Part IV you'll learn to put the concepts and exercises about energy, health, and illness into a more spiritual context by looking at the connection between physical well-being and higher levels of development.

Part IV

Beyond Physical Health

CHAPTER 15

You've Got Soul—
Physical Health,
Spiritual Development,
and Beyond . . .

"When I first heard of Pranic Healing, I was employed as a licensed physical therapist assistant who worked with chronic-pain patients. I went to class hoping simply to learn some new healing techniques that would help my patients, nearly all of whom get little relief from most traditional medical treatments. But not only did I acquire new healing techniques that did help my patients tremendously, I learned a new way to become spiritually closer and connected to God. This was totally unexpected. As an ordained lay minister in my church and someone who for years had completed prayer journals, I felt that my spiritual life and relationship with God were already very fulfilling. Yet what I learned from Master Co, especially how to perform the Meditation on Twin Hearts, was beyond any spiritual experience I had ever had. During this meditation I felt a oneness and connectedness to God that I had never felt before. I could actually feel God's love pouring over me and through me, opening my heart to respond to this love. Practicing this meditation daily gave me a new and powerful awareness of how we are truly instruments of the Divine.

"I had also been doing service for years in my church and community—or so I thought. After practicing this meditation and studying the teachings of Grandmaster Choa and Master Co, I came to see how limited my understanding of service really was. I now fully realize that 'it is in giving that we receive.' My original desire was to learn simply how to heal my patients more effectively. But now, my life is more spiritually—and even financially—abundant than I ever imagined because of the teachings I have learned."

—KIM FANTINI, BELLEVILLE, ILLINOIS

In this final chapter we put physical health and energy into a spiritual context. It's a natural next step for many who explore physical health through alternative or esoteric methods, and it's a particularly appropriate next step for those exploring energy-based healing.

Let's begin with the Dissociation Meditation. Take your time with it. Let your imagination go, and pay attention to your feelings. It's simple to perform, but it can have a dramatic effect on how you view your body, your mind, and your physical health. It may be easier for you to read through the exercise first, so that you are able to do it without having to read each step.

EXERCISE 15–A: **Dissociation Meditation**

1. Sit down in a darkened room, close your eyes, and go through your physical relaxation routine. Perform seven cycles of pranic breathing. Be aware of your whole body.

2. Put your attention on your feet and legs for several seconds. Continue pranic breathing, and then see and feel them disappear.

3. Put your attention on your waist, chest, and torso for several seconds. Continue pranic breathing, and then see and feel them disappear.

4. Put your attention on your hands and arms for several seconds. Continue pranic breathing, and then see and feel them disappear.

5. Put your attention on your head for several seconds. Continue pranic breathing, and then see and feel your head disappear.

6. Perform several cycles of pranic breathing as you are aware of your body "not being there."

7. Silently say, "I am not the body; I exist independently of the body." Be still for about 30 seconds.

8. Visualize a reddish-pink silhouette or outline of your physical body.

9. Silently say, "This is my emotional body. It contains any emotions that I have ever created or experienced. It allows me to feel and experience emotions and feelings, but it is not me."

10. See it fading and vaporizing into nothingness.

11. Silently say, "I am not the body, I am not the emotions. I exist independently of the physical and emotional bodies." Be still for about 30 seconds.

12. Visualize a bluish-yellowish silhouette or outline of your physical body.

13. Silently say, "This is my mental body. It contains any thoughts that I have ever created or experienced. It allows me to think and experience thoughts and ideas, but it is not me."

14. See it fading and vaporizing into nothingness.

15. Silently say, "I am not the body, I am not the emotions, nor the thoughts. I exist independently of the physical, emotional, and mental bodies." Be still for about 30 seconds.

16. Silently say, "I am not the body; the body is a vehicle of the soul. I am not my emotions or my thoughts; they are just products of the soul. I am not even the mind. The mind is just the instrument of the soul. I am the soul! I am a being of Divine Intelligence, Divine Love, and Divine Power. I am connected to God. I am one with God. I am one with All. I am the Soul!" Be still for 3 to 5 minutes and simply let go.

17. Slowly open your eyes, take several pranic breaths, and stretch.

As you perform this exercise, you realize that "you" are not your body. Nor are "you" your thoughts or emotions. Even if your body and thoughts were to disappear physically, not just figuratively, "you" would remain. This "you" or "I am" that you've been in touch with in this meditation is your soul.

The soul is a spark from the universal flame, which some call God. God puts forth this portion of himself, which then incarnates, or takes a body, in the lower plane, the earth. As an extension of God, our soul is in a state of permanent health, a state of unchanging, prolonged awareness and peace. We may not be consciously aware of it, but we inherently know that this state of peace resides within us.

As we seek health, success, and happiness in the physical world, we are often oblivious to how close *true* health, success, and happiness are, because we don't look inward. But when we become aware of the limitations of our physical body and the imperfections of the material world—as we must inevitably—our innate knowledge of this inner state of peace and health is stirred. This is called *spiritual restlessness*.

There are many ways spiritual restlessness is awakened. It is commonly prompted by a life crisis, such as a reversal of fortune or tragedy that is difficult to explain—for example, disastrous material loss or the death of someone close. It is often felt when we have a premature brush with mortality ourselves, or when we near the end of our life and seek to put things in order. Or, we may feel it after we attain our worldly goals—success, fame, prosperity, or in the case of our focus here, physical health—and then find ourselves wondering if "that's all there is." It may arise simply as a result of exploring physical health through alternative or esoteric practices, as you are doing with this book. Or it may be awakened naturally in those who are particularly sensitive or spiritually developed. Regardless of how we come to this awareness, we all have within us this intrinsic need to "return to the source," to have contact with our soul to access that inner peace and health.

Inner Peace Amid Chaos

It is said that years ago a certain spiritual master held a contest among his students to see who could draw the best representation of complete inner peace. Most of the paintings were of vast mountains with snow-capped peaks standing silent and majestic, or calm lakes, reflecting perfectly the trees around them in a glass-smooth surface, or dark forests of fir trees, so dense and quiet you could hear a leaf falling to the ground. But one student painted a scene of a violent storm with thunder cracking and lightning flashing while rain poured down in torrents, feeding a waterfall that crashed down a mountain. The student also painted, behind that waterfall, in a dark, dry crack that extended deep into the rock of the mountain, a single live branch on which sat a small bird's nest. In that deep crevasse in the mountain, the mother bird and her babies were dry, safe, and quiet while the storm raged around them.

Which of the pictures most accurately reflects the physical world and our quest for calm in a world of turmoil? Which of the pictures best portrays our search for inner stillness amid the ceaseless, disordered chatter of our "monkey mind"? This is the essence of our inherent desire to make contact with the soul: We need to know that there is order or meaning in a disorderly or meaningless world, that there is a place of inner peace amid this chaos.

The formula through which we tap into this inner peace is simple: "Flush out the channel," or open the spiritual cord that runs from the crown chakra to the soul; and "tune in" to the right frequency, by cultivating stillness and awareness during meditation. When the mind is still and the body energetically clean, the soul can reach down and make contact with us, which gives us access to inner peace.

The six steps in this book help you follow that formula. Regulating and clearing negative emotions, daily pranic breathing, and energetic hygiene work together to flush out your channel. The Mindfulness Meditation and the Meditation on Twin Hearts give you the right frequency you need to achieve stillness and awareness. The energy-manipulation techniques and energy-generation exercises give you the physical health and level of overall energy to pursue a higher path.

PHYSICAL HEALTH AND SPIRITUAL DEVELOPMENT

If you decide to intensify your practice and move beyond physical health to more spiritual matters, there are six other areas of inquiry you must consider. All are advanced concepts and deserve more discussion than we devote to them here. But this section gives you enough information to begin incorporating them into your personal plan for physical and spiritual development, if you wish. They are:

1. Increased need for purification and energetic hygiene
2. Proper attitude and respect for the teachings and sources of energy
3. Service
4. Karma
5. Tithing
6. Kundalini syndrome

Increased Need for Purification and Energetic Hygiene

A finely tuned race car is more prone to mechanical problems than the family station wagon, and the well-conditioned professional athlete suffers more muscle pulls and strains than the casual jogger. Pushing a machine or the physical body to higher performance levels while increasing the intensity and frequency of training brings with it greater risks of breakdown. Similarly, the more you develop your personal supply of prana, and the more you move onto a path that includes spiritual as well as physical development, the more sensitive you will become to "energetic breakdowns," or contamination through diet, words, thoughts, deeds, personal habits, and personal interactions.

Here's another way to look at it. If a boulder rolls down a mountain hill and blocks part of a seldom-used road, it will cause a problem for the few people who use that road, but it won't create a massive traffic tie-up. If someone drops a suitcase in the middle of a heavily traveled interstate that cuts through a major city, however, traffic will be slowed down and backed up, possibly for miles. You are learning to convert your energy channels from small country roads to superhighways. The traffic on them will increase from the occasional slow-moving pick-up truck to constant daily travel by thousands of high-speed cars. You need to keep that freeway, your energy channels, as clear as possible of obstructions.

Higher-level energy work requires a higher level of energetic hygiene.

Proper Attitude and Respect for the Teachings and Sources of Energy

Let's illustrate this with an experiment that demonstrates how attitude affects your supply of prana and your health.

EXERCISE 15–B: **Proper Attitude**

It's easier to do this exercise with two people, but you can perform it on a visualization of yourself. Begin with your standard warm-up.

1. Stand to the side of your subject at comfortable scanning distance. Or if you're scanning a visualization of yourself, imagine yourself within scanning distance, as if you were going to obtain an energetic baseline.

2. Get an energetic baseline reading, or do a quick scan at several points to establish the general depth and strength of the aura.

3. Now, have the subject either say aloud or think, with intent, these words (if you're scanning yourself, you can say or think them): "This energy I am generating is my own and no one else's. I alone am responsible for increasing and generating this prana, and I owe no responsibility to anyone else or any higher being for how I use it."

4. Rescan. You should find your hand moving in as the aura shrinks. If you scan as the words are spoken, your hand should sink in dramatically.

5. Now have the subject say aloud (or think) with intent these words: "I am truly grateful for the gift of this prana. I appreciate that I am able to use this divine spiritual energy to heal myself and further my spiritual development, and also to help others and contribute to the betterment of humanity."

6. As these words are spoken, you should feel a substantial strengthening of the energy aura.

To move beyond using prana only for physical health, you must cultivate a deep sense of gratitude for this universal energy and its source. Healers with a highly developed visual awareness can see that people with the proper "attitude of gratitude" have clean, balanced chakras, with the upper chakras (heart, throat, and head) slightly larger than the lower chakras (basic, navel, and solar plexus). This is the ideal proportion, for it means that the upper chakras, which control our higher or more spiritual impulses, are governing our lower chakras, which control our lower or more worldly impulses. Our higher impulses include characteristics such as lovingkindness, generosity, unselfishness, mercy, and wisdom. We employ these traits outwardly, toward other people, to create good in the world. Our lower impulses include self-preservation, desire for prosperity, and success. We employ these traits to create good for ourselves. This doesn't mean it is *wrong* to desire to do good for ourselves. We do need to take care of ourselves. It's just that these desires need to be tempered by higher impulses such as wisdom, mercy, and lovingkindness. Otherwise they lead to selfishness.

People who are less spiritually developed frequently hold the belief that this energy is theirs to use primarily for themselves. They feel no sense of gratitude for this gift of prana and are selfish, prideful, or arrogant. Their chakras are dirty and unbalanced, with lower chakras substantially larger than upper chakras. Their aura's energy is also more gross and less refined.

An attitude of humility and gratitude for the gift of this divine spiritual energy increases your body's ability to assimilate prana. An attitude of excessive pride or selfishness and an inability to attribute the energy properly to its source will reduce your ability to absorb prana, thereby shrinking your energy field, further evidence of the toxicity of negative emotions.

Service

Service means being generous in every way you can, in appreciation for life and this bountiful prana that sustains all life. You can be generous with many things: love, blessings, time, knowledge, support, talents, and resources. Being in service to the world helps you maintain the proper attitude of gratitude and humility.

Here's a quick exercise that demonstrates why we need to give back for receiving this gift of prana:

Take a reasonably deep breath, about half your lung capacity, and hold it. Without exhaling, breathe in again and hold it. While still holding your breath, inhale again to your full capacity and hold it. What would happen if you didn't exhale? Eventually, you're forced to exhale. You have to, or you'd be very uncomfortable.

Just as you can't continually breathe in without breathing out, you can't draw in and utilize this gift of spiritual energy without giving something back, in some form of service. The prana builds up in your energy body and creates congestion; you become uncomfortable. It is an abundant universe, and you are free to learn how to draw in and use prana for your own personal health and spiritual development. But as you use and accumulate it and learn more about it—which is to say, as you *develop spiritually*—you take on a responsibility to pass it along in the form of service, good works, and regular practice of positive virtues.

Here is an example. There are two basic ways to lift weights. Bodybuilders engage in a routine that focuses on building specific muscle groups in order to look good. They lift lower-than-maximum weights at a slow or measured pace with many repetitions to build that lean bodybuilder look. This routine doesn't necessarily translate into high performance in athletics, but bodybuilders are judged not on what they do but how they *look*.

Powerlifters and athletes in training for specific sports, on the other hand, perform weight-lifting routines designed to build up what they call functional strength. Their workouts are designed to help them perform their athletic movements better. For example, football linemen lift very heavy weights in short, explosive movements with few repetitions. These exercises build the specific muscle groups they use in their competitive endeavors, and they mimic the movements used on the football field. Powerlifters and football players are judged not on how they look but on what they do, how they *perform*.

In accumulating prana, you are building "spiritual muscles." You can use them solely for your own benefit, to "look good." Or, you can use them to develop spiritual "functional strength," which helps you perform service and good works, which ultimately return to you.

One very good way to offer service is to perform healings on other people. This form of service can also benefit you directly and quickly, for when you work on someone else's physical ailments, you often experience healing yourself. There are two reasons for this: First, the prana that you draw in passes through your energetic anatomy and has a cleansing and energizing effect on you. Second, you build up good karma with your service to another person in need. So in healing others, you may find yourself healed too. As Grandmaster Choa is fond of saying, "You cannot hold a torch to light another's path without illuminating your own."

After performing Pranic Healing on another person, students frequently report that they feel uplifted and energized. Kathleen Foronjy says she feels "cleaner and [more] peaceful in my heart." Tiffany Cano and many others experience that their own chakras become "larger and more activated." Scott Alexander says that, even after practicing Pranic Healing for two years, "one of the most surprising things I have noticed is how I feel after providing a treatment for someone. I feel really calm, quiet, centered, and totally energized. It is like I have been given a gift of extra life force for just being of service."

In short, if you are interested solely in your own health, you certainly will make progress using the six steps you've learned here, and it will likely be dramatic, as long as you're not selfish or prideful. But if you're interested in what might be called the overall health of the world—if you regularly and generously give back in service to show appreciation for your ability to generate and use this divine prana—you experience more rapid increases in your physical health and your spiritual development.

There are many other ways to offer service besides providing physical healings. For instance, a number of Pranic Healing practitioners in and around Los Angeles have begun a homeless feeding program called Feed Your Soul. Lindsay Hirsch-Adlam, a new Pranic Healing student, has been involved with the effort since its inception, and has found the experience moving and motivating. "The change in my life has been substantial," she says. "I feel a greater connection with humankind. I also feel more able to help those in need around me, as it has opened up a channel that allows me to be more proactive in helping others. We all think about helping others, but once we start actually doing it there is a snowball effect; we get into the habit of helping. The energetic effects of performing this service include significant growth and strength of all my chakras, and especially my hand chakras."

Here is another take on the importance of service and giving from ancient teachings. Taoist sages explained that nature is governed by a law of cycles. These cycles manifest in the world in such dual-faceted principles as light and dark, inhaling and exhaling, drawing in energy and putting forth energy, and giving and receiving. Each of the two elements in the pair is defined in relation to its opposite, and both are necessary for balance or equilibrium in the world. You can't have light without dark, and as you saw earlier, you can't inhale without exhaling. When there is an imbalance—too much or not enough of one or the other—this law is broken, and it creates a problem that nature will correct. Thus, if someone wants only to receive but not give, eventually nature will see to it that the person is unable to receive. Alternatively, if someone wants always to give but never receive—the person is unable to accept graciously—eventually nature will see to it that the person is unable to give. To be properly balanced and to be in harmony with natural law, we must be able both to give and to receive. Giving or providing service, whether you are offering love, time, money, or talent, creates a vacuum that enables you to receive more of what you gave. Receiving graciously, in turn, replenishes you and enables you to give even more. Service is thus part of the natural cycle of the universe and an important part of your physical, psychological, spiritual, and even financial health.

The principle of service is summarized perfectly in the simple phrase "As you give, so shall you receive."

Karma

Karma is the unbreakable cosmic law of cause and effect. It maintains that if you perform bad actions or deeds, they return to you in some negative form. Likewise, if you perform good actions or deeds, they too return, but in some positive or favorable form. Karma is a term that has become popularized to mean "what goes around comes around," or to refer to some type of "cosmic justice system." Yet karma does function exactly like that.

Some question the validity of karma as a universal principle because they do not always see the law applied in the way they'd like or expect. They observe that many "bad" people are outwardly successful or happy, while many "good" or "innocent" people are suffering. But we often lack the wisdom and insight to see through the appearances of this physical world. Just because we don't see immediate punishment in this world for "bad" deeds and immediate reward for "good" doesn't invalidate the law of karma. The law of karma is unbreakable and unchangeable.

Karma and Physical Health

Any discussion of karma naturally leads to questions about its effect on health. If all our thoughts and actions come back to us in some form, is there a causal relationship between a health problem and some action we have taken or not taken? The answer is, . . . possibly. With physiological cause and effect, it's easy to see the relationship. If you have a family history of heart disease and diabetes and yet you are overweight, have high blood pressure, and refuse to make more healthful life choices, you are likely to reap the consequences, or karma, of your actions: Heart attack, stroke, circulation and eyesight problems are just a few possible complications.

Some health conditions can be due to "cosmic" cause and effect. For instance, in esoteric philosophy, it has long been held that if you cause pain to fellow human beings or are cruel to animals, you may develop some type of ailment that causes you great pain. Other health problems are believed to result from bad actions such as lying, cheating, and stealing.

How can you tell if your health problem has a karmic connection? More important, how do you remedy it? If you practice the routine in this book regularly and have had success with self-healing, yet are unable to relieve yourself of a problem, your condition could be related to karma. You determine this through self-examination, the self-awarenes exercise (Exercise 3–A), and meditation. It isn't as mysterious and difficult as you might think. Most people who engage in this self-analysis develop a sense or gut feel that the problem is or isn't due to cosmic karmic causes. Here's a quick routine for determining karmic involvement in a health problem:

1. Start with the Mindfulness Meditation.
2. After 5 minutes, place your awareness on your health problem.
3. Formulate in your mind a question such as, "Has this condition been caused by any action or inaction on my part that I need to resolve?"
4. Let go, and return to being aware and mindful.

You may get an answer in that meditation. You may get an answer later in the day, or the next day. Or, you may have to meditate on it for several days. The answer may come to you in an indirect, surprising, or symbolic way. (Remember, the unconscious mind doesn't always communicate verbally.)

Resolving Karmically Related Health Problems

There are three steps to follow:

1. *Learn your lessons.* You need to determine the cause and correct it. Make reparations to the extent that you can. For instance, if you determine that your neck spasms were caused in part because you were a "pain in the neck" to your parents when you were growing up, you need to make amends for your actions. You might begin by sincerely apologizing to them and asking for forgiveness. If you've stolen something, begin by making restitution.
2. *Practice the law of forgiveness.* If you intend to seek forgiveness for some past action or inaction, you need to practice forgiveness with others who may have hurt you. As it is written in Matthew 6:14: "For if you forgive men when they sin against you, your heavenly Father will also forgive you." This step might include releasing any grudges you hold against someone who wronged or hurt you. Forgiveness has a powerful cleansing effect on the front and back solar plexus chakras. Some people hold so much anger and resentment in these chakras that without forgiveness, no matter how much these chakras are cleansed, they generate the dirty energy again.
3. *Practice the law of mercy.* In order to develop your spiritual muscles and demonstrate humility, you must be merciful and tolerant in your current personal interactions. In Matthew 5:7, we read: "Blessed are the merciful for they will be shown mercy." This step might include being less harsh and judgmental in your general dealings with people.

These steps to atone for or "work out" bad karma should be done directly, if possible. If you've hurt someone, apologize in person if you can. Similarly, if you've stolen something, make restitution to the person from whom you've stolen if you can. Direct restitution isn't always possible, however. Perhaps the person you hurt or stole from is dead, or you've lost contact with them. If so, you can also perform these steps symbolically. For instance, simply invoke, perform several cycles of pranic breathing, picture the person you wronged in front of you, and express a sincere apology for your actions. You can take the same figurative steps in releasing a grudge or hard feelings against people. You can also work out karma for theft by making a donation to a charitable organization.

Finally, while many emphasize the "negative" or "punishment" aspect of the law of karma, there is a better and more positive way to view it: as a means to build the future you want. When you fully understand the implications of the law of karma, you are empowered. You realize you can take action to create new "causes" or "seeds" in your physical, psychological, spiritual—and even financial—life, and reap the "effects" of the seeds that you sow.

Tithing

An especially powerful method of utilizing the law of karma to improve your life, and a very effective way to neutralize negative karma, is tithing. In its strict dictionary definition, *tithing* means giving a tenth of one's earnings to the church. In a more general sense, however, it means contributing whatever amount of money you can to good and worthy causes.

The esoteric principle behind tithing stems from the law of karma: "You reap what you sow." As you give generously of yourself and your resources, that generosity will be returned to you in kind. If you view your karma as your "cosmic financial statement," you might say that tithing gives you a way to build up a "positive balance." If you donate $100 to a charity, at some point in the future $100 in good karma credit or value will return to you. This karmic credit may take the form of money, success in some venture, good health for you or your family, general good luck, or something else of comparable value that you may need or want.

Tithing is used in a number of health- and spiritually related ways:

- To demonstrate gratitude for the blessings of life and energy.
- To demonstrate proper attitude and humility.
- To build up good karma credits.
- To atone for past bad actions or to work out bad karma (particularly if you are unable to reconcile with someone in person).
- To help accelerate self-healing of ailments that are at least partially attributable to bad karma.
- To plant the seeds of good health, happiness, prosperity, and spiritual fulfillment.

How to Tithe

If you wish to make tithing a regular part of your health- and spiritual-development routine, here are some guidelines:

Amount. Ten percent of your income, after taxes, is the "standard" recommendation; however, this is not feasible for everyone. You can start with a smaller percentage and work you way up to 10 percent.

Proper tithing beneficiaries. It is good to tithe to organizations that help people in great need. Any organization that helps the homeless, disaster victims, or those suffering from serious illnesses is good. But you may also want to tithe to further a particular cause, especially if you are trying to atone for a past wrongdoing or are asking for help in a particular area. Here are some examples:

- If you're atoning for selfish impulses or actions and you want to be more giving and generous, it might be good to donate to the Salvation Army or a rescue mission because they help people who are in great need.
- If you are addressing the karmic cause of a current health condition, it might be good to donate to an organization that raises funds for research in fighting that problem or something similar to it.
- If you were cruel to animals when you were a child, it might be good to make a donation to an animal shelter or rescue fund.

It is also good to give money or money equivalents (gifts) to people or organizations that have directly contributed to your physical, emotional, spiritual, or financial well-being. This includes churches, spiritual organizations, your parents, and your employees (if you own or run a business), to name just a few. This is a critical aspect of tithing that most teachings overlook. It shows gratitude for the blessings you have received.

Frequency. Some people tithe a full year in advance; others write checks monthly or every two or three months. There is no karmically best way to tithe with regard to frequency. It's more a matter of convenience and whether you wish to donate to many causes or a few. It's an individual decision.

Here is a sample tithing routine:

EXERCISE 15–C: *Tithing Routine*

1. Invoke for guidance and blessings.
2. Write a check for whatever amount you decide to the organization or person(s) of your choice.
3. Hold the check in your hands and say to yourself or aloud, with sincere intent, that you are grateful for the opportunity to serve, that you intend that this donation help as many

people as possible, and that you wish it to generate much good karma for you and your family (if applicable). Include in your prayer also your wish that this donation offset or "work out" any bad karma you may have incurred. Finally, if you have a specific cause, such as self-healing, simply add that you would like your donation to generate good karma that will be applied to your healing.

4. Then let go of the thought, mail the check, and forget about it.

You can decide if tithing fits in with your belief system, but the health and spiritual benefits of tithing can be profound; they go far beyond just the good feeling you get when you give to those in need.

Tithing and Healing

"My grandmother suffered two severe strokes that caused her brain stem to bleed, and she ended up in a coma. We performed Pranic Healing regularly, but she made only minor improvements. I then remembered what Grandmaster Choa taught about tithing and healing: If you want to save your own life or the life of a loved one, give to organizations that save people's lives. I brought to the hospital one envelope addressed to the local chapter of the Red Cross and another addressed to the national disaster relief chapter of the Red Cross. I asked my aunts to place $1,000 of my grandmother's money into each envelope. It had to be my grandmother's money, because the healing was for her. I then instructed them to decree that the money should be utilized to save people's lives and that the good karma generated by this donation should be applied to Grandmother's rapid recovery. After the giving, I scanned her and noticed that her energy level started to increase. Three days later, she opened her eyes!

"When tithing with a sincere intent was added to Pranic Healing, my grandmother, against medical odds, regained her mental functions and is now perfectly healthy!"

—*Master Stephen Co*

Kundalini Syndrome

Kundalini is a powerful energy that lies dormant near the base of the spine until it is stimulated through yogic postures and breathing exercises. It is related to but slightly different from prana. One of the main goals of some forms of yoga is to awaken the kundalini, so that practitioners can use it to power rapid spiritual development and enlightenment. But awakening kundalini can be a risky proposition. If done improperly, too soon, or without appropriate preparation, safeguards, or instruction, it can lead to numerous energetic disturbances and physical, emotional, and mental problems. Yogic literature is filled with first-person accounts of practitioners who awakened the kundalini unsafely and suffered insomnia, weakening of the body, serious health problems, uncontrolled negative emotions, and even hallucinations.

As you progress and increase the quantity and quality of your prana, you may find yourself occasionally experiencing a mild version of what energy masters call *kundalini syndrome*, which results from higher-voltage prana hitting a blockage in your energy body and creating congestion. Kundalini syndrome differs from a routine energy blockage in that it may manifest not only as a physical feeling, such as tightness or discomfort in the body, but also as a magnification of a negative character trait or a downturn in life circumstances. For example, you may feel strangely irritable or angry for no apparent reason. You may experience a financial, career, or personal reversal. Or you may have a stretch of just plain "bad luck" for which there is no apparent cause; nothing seems to work out right for you. Such abrupt changes in your life are due to stronger prana expediting the materialization of your karma. Serious students of high-level esoteric and energy practices view kundalini syndrome and the *karmic acceleration* that often accompanies it as part of the purification process they must undergo on the spiritual path. It's a way of more rapidly doing penance for past bad thoughts, words, and deeds and advancing spiritual growth.

The Pranic Healing routines presented in this book are designed to minimize the possibility of kundalini syndrome. The progressive nature of the exercises and the emphasis on energetic hygiene will help your energy development keep pace with your energetic cleanliness. If you follow the step-by-step instructions, the amount of energy you build should not exceed your body's ability to accommodate it. Some people who practice Pranic Healing still do experience kundalini syndrome, however. If you do, the remedy is simple:

- Stop energy-generation exercises and meditations temporarily.
- Go on a cleaner diet: no meat or fish until you stabilize.
- Take a salt bath daily.
- Perform general sweeping and specific sweeping of affected parts daily.
- Release the excess or blocked energies by blessing the earth with your outstretched hands, just as you did in the Meditation on Twin Hearts. This alone will induce a sense of inner peace and relief from congestion.

That should take care of kundalini syndrome within a couple of days.

WILL I BE "STUCK" ON THIS PATH?

As students become aware of the larger spiritual context of their physical health and the depth of this work, some wonder if they will be "stuck" on the spiritual path if they decide to pursue it. They are concerned that they will have to give up aspects of "normal" life, such as eating certain foods or interacting with old friends. When you begin to incorporate these six steps for greater health and energy into your life—and even if you adopt some of the advanced concepts in this chapter—most assuredly you will *not* be entering a path from which you can't escape or deviate. We've said throughout this book—and we say it in our classes—that as you learn the material and the exercises, make up your own mind as to whether they're beneficial for you. Let your experiences with them, as well as your personal belief system, dictate to what degree you wish to make these teachings part of your life. Many people have realized that these practices give them the ability to make more effective choices as they seek more control over their life, their energy, and their health.

The teachings that underlie the routines presented here are incredibly rich, and this book on physical healing just scratches their surface. For those with a hunger for additional information, there is much more to learn.

ADDING THESE ADVANCED CONCEPTS TO YOUR ROUTINE

If you wish to add these components to your routine, here are some guidelines:

Increased purification: More diligent adherence to an energetically clean diet, more regular practice of emotional regulation.

Proper attitude and respect: Begin *every* practice with a sincere invocation.

Service: This is an individual decision, but consider performing three hours of service a week.

Karma: Review regularly during meditation your past thoughts, words, and deeds; make amends where necessary.

Tithing: As with service, tithing is an individual decision. Contribute what you can to appropriate organizations each month.

*   *   *

You now have a whole new way of looking at the world and your health. You have an incredible array of tools and exercises to increase your energy and heal yourself. But your real personal health work is just beginning. You must apply the principles and practice the exercises regularly.

Stay well.

SOURCES AND NOTES

Chapter 1

1. Energetic anatomy, pp. 14–21, from *Miracles Through Pranic Healing* (Grandmaster Choa Kok Sui), and Basic Pranic Healing course.

2. Energetic template material, pp. 26–27, from *The Body Electric: Electromagnetism and the Foundation of Life* (Becker).

Chapter 2

1. Part of functional ailments discussion, pp. 31–33, from *Phantom Illness: Shattering the Myth of Hypochondria* (Cantor).

2. Part of mind-body connection discussion, pp. 33–34, from interview with Dr. Candace Pert in *Healing and the Mind* (Moyers).

3. Part of unconscious discussion, pp. 34–35, from Dr. Tad James' Neurolinguistic Programming Training Courses.

4. Negative emotions discussion, p. 36 and ff., from *Conscious Loving: The Journey to Co-Commitment*, and *At the Speed of Life: A New Approach to Personal Change Through Body-Centered Therapy* (both Hendricks).

5. Back pain discussion, pp. 37–38, from *Healing Back Pain: The Mind-Body Connection* (Sarno).

6. Part of unconscious mind discussion, pp. 40–41, from *Answer Cancer* (Parkhill).

Chapter 3

1. Direct clearing discussion, pp. 46–47, from *At the Speed of Life: A New Approach to Personal Change Through Body-Centered Therapy* (Hendricks).

2. Part of awareness discussion, pp. 48–49, from *Meditation* (Easwaren) and *Full Catastrophe Living: Using the Wisdom of Your Body and Mind to Face Stress, Pain, and Illness* (Kabat-Zinn).

3. Direct clearing discussion, p. 49, from Dr. Tad James' Neurolinguistic Programming Training Courses.

4. Part of clearing emotions discussion, pp. 50–54, from *At the Speed of Life: A New Approach to Personal Change Through Body-Centered Therapy* (Hendricks).

5. Part of higher-level thinking discussion, pp. 54–58, from Dr. Tad James' Neurolinguistic Programming Training Courses.

Chapter 4

1. Pranic breathing and related breathing techniques (exclusive of Exercises 4-A and 4-C), from Third Session, Modules 3.01.00–3.02.00, Grandmaster Choa Kok Sui Pranic Healing Course, Instructors Manual, 3rd ed., 1995.

2. Exercise 4-A, pp. 72–75, from *The Art of Chi Kung: Making the Most of Your Vital Energy* (Wong Kiew Kit).

3. Exercise 4-C, pp. 76–77, from *Conscious Breathing: Breathwork for Health, Stress Release, and Personal Mastery* (Hendricks).

4. "Master Breathing Technique," p. 77, from *Kosher Yoga* (Schutz and de Schaps).

Chapters 5 and 6

1. Scanning instruction, exercises, and techniques, from *Miracles Through Pranic Healing*, Basic Pranic Healing course, Pranic Self-Healing course, and Third Session, Module 3.03.00, Grandmaster Choa Kok Sui Pranic Healing Course, Instructors Manual, 3rd ed., 1995.

Chapter 7

1. Sweeping instruction, exercises, and techniques, from *Miracles Through Pranic Healing*, Basic Pranic Healing course, Pranic Self-Healing course, and Second Session, Module 2.06.00, Grandmaster Choa Kok Sui Pranic Healing Course, Instructors Manual, 3rd ed., 1995.

Chapter 8

1. Energizing instruction, exercises, and techniques, from *Miracles Through Pranic Healing*, Basic Pranic Healing course, Advanced Pranic Healing course, Pranic Self-Healing course, and private teachings from Grandmaster Choa Kok Sui.

Chapter 9

1. Use of color instruction, exercises, and techniques, from *Advanced Pranic Healing* (Grandmaster Choa Kok Sui), Advanced Pranic Healing course, Pranic Self-Healing course, and First Session, Modules 1.04.00–1.05.00, Grandmaster Choa Kok Sui Pranic Healing Course, Instructors Manual, 3rd ed., 1995.

Chapter 10

1. Energetic hygiene instruction, exercises and techniques (exclusive of Exercises 10-C, 10-I, and 10-J), from Basic Pranic Healing course, Advanced Pranic Healing course, and Pranic Self-Healing course.

2. Exercise 10-C, pp. 183–184, from Psychic Self-Defense course.

3. Exercises 10-I, pp. 191–192, and 10-J, pp. 193–194, from Arhatic Yoga Preparatory course.

Chapter 11

1. Basic concentration, awareness, and mindfulness instruction, material, and exercises, pp. 200–208, from *Meditations for Soul Realization* (Grandmaster Choa Kok Sui), and Meditations for Soul Realization course.

2. Meditation on Twin Hearts and related material, pp. 208–216, from *Meditations for Soul Realization*, Meditations for Soul Realization course, and Arhatic Yoga Preparatory course.

Chapter 12

1. Basic energy-generation instruction and concepts from Arhatic Yoga Preparatory course and private teachings from Grandmaster Choa Kok Sui.

2. Modified Tibetan Yogic Exercises, pp. 224–230, from Longevity course.

3. Modified Mentalphysics Exercises, pp. 231–242, from Fourth Session, Pranic Self-Healing course.

Chapter 13

1. Self-Healing Guide, from *Advanced Pranic Healing*, and *Advanced Pranic Healing* Instructors Manual.

Chapter 15

1. Dissociation Meditation, from World Pranic Healers Convention, 2000.

2. Higher-level spiritual instruction and concepts—proper attitude, service, tithing, karma, kundalini syndrome—from Arhatic Yoga Preparatory course, Arhatic Yoga review course, 2000, and private teachings from Grandmaster Choa Kok Sui.

FOR FURTHER REFERENCE

For More Information on Pranic Healing Products and Classes:

U.S. Pranic Healing Center
The American Institute of Asian Studies, LLC
3873 Schaefer Ave., Suite A
Chino, CA 91710
(888) 470-5656
www.pranichealing.com

Classes offered include:

- Basic Pranic Healing
- Advanced Pranic Healing
- Pranic Psychotherapy
- Pranic Crystal Healing
- Meditations for Soul Realization
- Pranic Psychic Self-Defense

These higher-level classes are offered exclusively by Grandmaster Choa Kok Sui at select locations around the world:

- Arhatic Yoga
- Pranic Feng Shui
- Kriyashakti (materialization of goals and increased prosperity)
- Higher Clairvoyance

For more information on material and concepts in this book, log on to *http://www.YourHands CanHealYou.com,* or call 1-888-9-HEAL YOU. Sign up on our e-mail list for updates on Pranic Healing.

Books

Bailey, Alice. *Esoteric Healing*. New York: Lucis Publishing Co., 1984.

_____. *Ponder On This*. New York: Lucis Publishing Co., 1980.

Becker, Robert, M.D. *The Body Electric: Electromagnetism and the Foundation of Life*. New York: William Morrow, 1987.

Cantor, Carla, and Brian Fallon. *Phantom Illness: Shattering the Myth of Hypochondria*. New York: Houghton Mifflin, 1996.

Choa Kok Sui, Grandmaster. *Advanced Pranic Healing: A Practical Manual on Color Pranic Healing*. Chino, CA: Institute for Inner Studies Publishing, 2000.

_____. *The Ancient Science and Art of Pranic Crystal Healing*. Chino, CA: Institute for Inner Studies Publishing, 1998.

_____. *Meditations for Soul Realization*. Chino, CA: Institute for Inner Studies Publishing, 2000.

_____. *Miracles Through Pranic Healing*. Nevada City, CA: Blue Dolphin Publishing, 2000.

_____. *Practical Psychic Self-Defense for Home and Office*. Chino, CA: Institute for Inner Studies Publishing, 1999.

_____. *Pranic Psychotherapy*. Chino, CA: Institute for Inner Studies Publishing, 2000.

Dingle, Edwin J. *Breaths That Renew Your Life*. Yucca Valley, CA: Institute of Mentalphysics, 1976.

Easwaran, Eknath. *Meditation: A Simple Eight-Point Program for Translating Spiritual Ideals into Daily Life*. Berkeley, CA: Nilgiri, 1991.

Hendricks, Gay, Ph.D. *Conscious Breathing: Breathwork for Health, Stress Release, and Personal Mastery*. New York: Bantam, 1995.

Hendricks, Gay, Ph.D., with Kathlyn Hendricks. *At the Speed of Life: A New Approach to Personal Change Through Body-Centered Therapy*. New York: Bantam, 1994.

_____. *Conscious Loving: The Journey to Co-Commitment*. New York: Bantam, 1992.

Kabat-Zinn, Jon, Ph.D. *Full Catastrophe Living: Using the Wisdom of Your Body and Mind to Face Stress, Pain, and Illness*. New York: Delta, 1990.

Kelder, Peter, and Bernie S. Siegel, M.D. *Ancient Secret of the Fountain of Youth*. New York: Doubleday, 1998.

Kilham, Christopher S. *The Five Tibetans*. Rochester, VT: Healing Arts Press, 1994.

Leadbeater, C.W. *The Inner Life*. Wheaton, IL: Theosophical Publishing House, 1996.

Long, Max Freedom. *The Secret Science at Work*. Marina Del Rey, CA: DeVorss & Co., 1953.

_____. *The Secret Science Behind Miracles*. Marina Del Rey, CA: DeVorss & Co., 1948.

Luk, Charles (Lu K'uan Yu). *The Secrets of Chinese Meditation*. York Beach, ME: Samuel Weiser; and London: Rider & Co., 1969.

_____. *Taoist Yoga: The Alchemy of Immortality*. York Beach, ME: Samuel Weiser; and London: Rider & Co., 1973.

Moyers, Bill. *Healing and the Mind*. New York: Doubleday, 1993.

Parkhill, Stephen. *Answer Cancer*. Fort Lauderdale: Omni Hypnosis, 2000.

Pelletier, Kenneth. *Mind As Healer, Mind As Slayer: A Holistic Approach to Preventing Stress Disorders*. New York: Delta, 1992.

Pert, Candace, Ph.D. *Molecules of Emotion: Why You Feel the Way You Feel*. New York: Simon & Schuster, 1999.

Sarno, John E., M.D. *Healing Back Pain: The Mind-Body Connection*. New York: Warner Books, 1991.

_____. *The Mindbody Prescription: Healing the Body, Healing the Pain*. New York: Warner Books, 1999.

Schutz, Albert L., and Hilda W. de Schaps. *Kosher Yoga*. Goleta, CA: Quantal Publishing, 1983.

Selye, Hans. *The Stress of Life*. New York: McGraw-Hill Professional Publishing, 1978.

Siegel, Bernie S., M.D. *Love, Medicine and Miracles: Lessons Learned About Self-Healing from a Surgeon's Experience with Exceptional Cancer Patients*. New York: Harper, 1990.

Slater, Wallace. *Raja Yoga*. Wheaton, IL: Theosophical Publishing House, 1992.

Wong Kiew Kit. *The Art of Chi Kung: Making the Most of Your Vital Energy*. Boston: Element Books, 1993.

Yogananda, Paramahansa. *Autobiography of a Yogi*. Los Angeles: Self-Realization Fellowship, 1946.

Products

Internal Cleansing

Colon Cleanse®
Health Plus, Inc.
13837 Magnolia Ave.
Chino, CA 91710
(800) 822-6225
www.healthplusinc.com

Green Foods, Blue-Green Algae

Green Magma
Green Foods Corporation
320 North Graves Ave.
Oxnard, CA 93030
(800) 777-4430
www.greenfoods.com

Klamath Blue Green
301 Old Stage Rd.
P.O. Box 1626
Mt. Shasta, CA 96067
(800) 327-1956
www.klamathbluegreen.com

Internal Cleansing

Colon Cleanse®
Health Plus, Inc.
13837 Magnolia Ave.
Chino, CA 91710
(800) 822-6225
www.healthplusinc.com

Oils, Incense

Soothe Your Soul
415 North Pacific Coast Hwy.
Redondo Beach, CA 90277
(310) 798-8445
(310) 372-2153

Vitamins,
General Supplements

Nature's Plus
Natural Organics
Headquarters
548 Broadhollow Rd.
Melville, NY 11747–3708
(800) 645-9500
www.naturesplus.com

Bee Products, Ginseng,
Other Energy-Generating
Supplements

Prince of Peace brand
Prince of Peace Enterprises
3536 Arden Rd.
Hayward, CA 94545
(800) 732-2328
www.popus.com

SELF-HEALING EXPERIENCE FORM

Use the following Self-Healing Experience form to let us know how these techniques worked for you. Send the form, via mail, fax, or e-mail, to:

U.S. Pranic Healing Center
The American Institute of Asian Studies
3873 Schaeffer Ave., Suite A
Chino, CA 91710
(888) 470-5656 (tel)/(909) 548-0886 (fax)
www.pranichealing.com

Name: _____ Age: _____ Telephone: _____

Address: _____

_____

Profession: _____

Health problem (describe it, how long you have had it, its effect on your life, traditional medical remedies you have tried, etc.):

_____

_____

_____

Self-healing treatment (what you did and for how long):

_____

_____

_____

Outcome (what the results were and how long it took):

_____

_____

May we quote you in a future book? _____ Yes_____ No _____ Ask me first

Signed: _____ Date: _____

INDEX

Abdomen, becoming aware of, 76–77

Abdominal breathing. *See* Pranic breathing

Abdominal pain, 37

Self-Sweeping with Colors, 167–168

Afternoon routine, 264

Air prana, 21, 22, 143, 193

Ajna (brows) chakra, 15, 16, 18, 19, 149, 169, 171, 183, 247

Alcohol, 115, 118, 127, 148, 194

Alcoholic drinks, 185

Alexander, Scott, 274

Alvarez, Karla, 124, 199–200

Amen, 193

Ancient Secrets of the Fountain of Youth (Kelder), 221

Anderson, Valerie, 203–204

Anger, 35, 38–39, 41, 53, 201

Animals, scanning, 92–93

Ankle rotations, 192

Anxieties, 29, 201

Appelgren, Laura, 222

Appetite control, 254

Armas, Alejandro, 77

Arthritis, 249–250

Asthma, 37, 250

At the Speed of Life: A New Approach to Personal Change Through Body-Centered Therapy (Hendricks), 46

Attitude, proper, 272–273, 282

Aura, 14–21, 21. *See also* Energetic anatomy

cleaning. *See* Sweeping

closing and Strengthening, 183–184

energizing. *See* Energizing

Autonomic nervous system (ANS), 33

Ayurveda, 11, 20

Back heart chakra, 15, 16, 18, 19

Back pain, 53, 130, 250–251

Back solar plexus chakra, 15, 16, 18, 19, 104, 105, 149, 167, 169–171

Back spleen chakra, 15, 17–19

Barley grass, 190

Basic chakra, 15, 17, 19, 20, 78, 149, 157–159, 172, 195

Bath, salt, 194–195

Becker, Robert, 26–27

Bee pollen, 190

Bee propolis, 190

Bio-energetics, 51

Bladder pain, 51

Bloating, 37

Blue-green algae, 190

Blue prana, 156, 157, 159, 160

Borman, Cynthia A., 3–4

Breathing, types of, 63–64

Bronchitis, 252–253

Buddha, 65

Burns, 251–252

Cano, Tiffany, 93, 274

Carpal tunnel, 252

Chakral baseline, 108

establishing, 108–109

variations, 109

Chakral technique, 143

Chakras, 13, 14. *See also* Self-healing; specific chakras

eleven major, 15–17

scanning for depth and strength, 98–100

scanning for width, 100–102

Chi, 10, 11, 28

Chi kung, 11–14, 28, 72, 142, 185, 205, 220

Choa Kok Sui, Grandmaster, 5, 9, 11–12, 77, 82, 123, 159, 193, 199, 208, 210, 218, 221, 274, 280

Chronic pain, 37–38

Clamping down, 37–39

Clapping, loud, 193

Clavicular breathing, 63, 74

Clawing, 124

Clean home and work environment, 193–194, 210

Cleanliness. *See* Sweeping

Cleansing. *See* Sweeping

Cleansing Breath, 238–239

Cleansing Physical Exercises, 191–192

Colds, 252–253

Colitis, 53

Collective unconscious, 34–35

Colon Cleanse, 187, 190

Colored pranas, 3, 12, 14, 155–175. *See also* Self-healing

Colored pranas (con't)
Advanced General Self-
Sweeping with Colors,
167–168
basics of using, 156
characteristics of, 157
checklist, 173–175
General Self-Sweeping with
Colors, 164–165
guidelines for safe and proper
use of, 159–161
Local Self-Sweeping with Col-
ors, 165–167
pregnant women and, 115,
160, 248
Self-Energizing with Colors—
Stress Relief, 169–171
sweeping and energizing with,
156, 158–159
testing pranic flow, 171–172
Visualization Practice with
Colors—Dual Colors
(Green-Blue), 163–164
Visualization Practice with
Colors—Single Colors,
162–163
Combing, 124–125
Compensatory hypertrophy, 27
Concentration, 200
Congestion, 13, 28, 42, 51, 107,
109. *See also* Sweeping
*Conscious Breathing: Breathwork for
Health* (Hendricks), 76
Conscious mind, 34
Conscious-unconscious dissocia-
tion, 48
Constipation, 37, 253
Cosmic consciousness, 207–208
Crown chakra, 15, 16, 18, 19, 66,
157, 159, 166, 208, 211, 212
Cutting cords, 115, 177, 180–182

Daily routine, 263–264
Davidovici, Arnon, 86–87, 161,
180–181
Denial, 36–37, 46
Depletion, 13, 28, 42, 107, 109.
See also Energizing

Depression, 23, 253–254
Diagnostic tests, 32
Diaphragm, 66–68
stretching and loosening, 70,
72–74, 96, 110
Diaphragmatic breathing, 64
Diarrhea, 37, 255
Diet, 184–191, 254
drinking water, cleaning and
energizing, 188
Energetically Cleaning Food,
187
herbs and supplements,
189–190
recommendations for energeti-
cally clean, 185–188
"Retroactive" Food Cleansing,
187–188
Differential diagnosis, 32
Dingle, Edwin J., 222
Direct clearing techniques, 46–47,
49–58, 96, 110
Dirty energy. *See* Sweeping
Dissociation Meditation, 268–270
Distracting, 46
Distributive sweeping, 13
Diverting, 46
Divine invocation, 143
Dozier, Barbara, 155
Drinking water, cleaning and ener-
gizing, 188—
Dual-colored pranas, 156

Earache, 254
Earth prana, 21, 22
Easwaren, Eknath, 207
Elbow, finger shake, 24, 85
Electric violet prana, 156, 157,
159, 160, 172, 194
Emotional contamination, 178
Emotional regulation, 178–184
Emotions, negative. *See* Negative
emotions and limiting
beliefs, clearing
Endocrine system, 33
Energetic anatomy, 9, 14–21, 41
basic components of, 14
chakras. *See* Chakras

Detecting Your Personal,
23–25, 84
meridians, 20–21
principal functions of, 15
Energetic baseline, 105–106, 149
establishing, 106–107
variations, 108
Energetic benefits of pranic
breathing, 68–70
Energetic hygiene, 12, 30, 47,
177–197, 223, 247
hecklist, 196–197
clean home and work environment, 193–194
diet, 184–191
emotional regulation, 178–184
increased need for, 271
keys to, 178
physical exercise, 191–192
salt, 194–196
Energetic template, scientific evidence of, 26–27
Energizing, 3, 12, 13, 20, 47,
114, 142–153, 189–190
checklist, 153–154
with colored pranas, 156,
158–159
Depleted Areas or Chakras of
Another Person Using Sim-
ple Projection, 148–150
Depleted Areas or Chakras of
Another Person Using
Water Pump Technique,
150–151
drinking water, 188
proper hand position for,
143–144
Self-Energizing Depleted Areas
or Chakras Using Water
Pump Technique, 151–152
Self-Energizing with Colors—
Stress Relief, 169–171
Simple Projection: Visualization Practice, 146–148
sweeping before, 143–144
Energy body. *See* Energetic
anatomy
Energy-generation exercises.
See Mentalphysics Exercises;

Tibetan Yogic Exercises
Energy manipulation. *See* Energizing; Scanning; Sweeping
Energy medicine, 10
    examples of, 11
    Pranic Healing compared to, 12–14
Eenvironmental contamination, 178
Epsom salts, 114, 194
Eucalyptus oil, 195
Exercise, 191–192, 205, 210
Expanded awareness, 207
External generation, 142
Eye rotations, 191
Eyestrain, 254

Fantini, Kim, 97, 267–268
Fear, 29, 36, 41, 201
Fever, 252–253
Fifth Tibetan Yogic Exercise, 229–230
Fight-or-flight response, 201
First Tibetan Yogic Exercise, 224–225
Fish, 184–186
Five Rites of Rejuvenation, The (Kelder), 221
Five Tibetans, The (Kilham), 221
Food. *See* Diet
Food poisoning, 255
Foods, energetically clean and dirty, 184–185
Forehead chakra, 15, 16, 18, 19
Forgiveness, 277
Foronjy, Kathleen, 274
Fourth Tibetan Yogic Exercise, 228–229
Fowl, 184
Front heart chakra, 15, 16, 18, 19, 153
Front solar plexus chakra, 15, 16, 18, 19, 98–102, 128–130, 136–137, 149, 167, 169, 170, 181, 182
Front spleen chakra, 15, 17–19
Fruits, 184–186
Full integration, state of, 47–49

Full visualization, 134
Functional boundaries, 35–36, 41
Functional channel, 20
Functional disorders, 31, 32, 37, 53

Garlic, 190
General Self-Scanning, 83, 110
    of arm, 87–90
General Self-Sweeping, 130–133
    with Colors, 164–165
    with Colors (Advanced), 167–168
    Dog-Paddle Routine, 131–133
    of Health Rays, 133–134
    10-Sweep Routine, 131
General Sweeping
    of Another Person, 117–122
    of Health Rays of Another Person, 123–125
Ginseng, 190
Glaucoma, 210
Goldfish, 27
Gold prana, 156
Goodwin, Paul, 35
Governor channel, 20
Grains, 184, 185
Grand Rejuvenation Breath, 239–240
Green-blue prana, 156, 157, 159, 163–164
Green foods, 190
Green prana, 156, 157, 159, 160, 162, 164–172, 194
Grounding, 207, 215
Ground prana, 21, 143
Growth hormones, 185
Guidera, Anthony, 151–152

Hand looseners, 192
Hand openers, 24, 84
Hand Sensitivity Exercise 1, 23–25, 84, 86, 87, 89, 90, 96, 110
Hand Sensitivity Exercise 2, 84–87, 89, 90, 96, 110
Harmonic Breath (Balancing

Breathing), 231–232
Healing state, 112
Health aura, 14, 21, 123
Heart chakra, 15, 16, 18, 84, 89, 90, 208, 210, 212
Hendricks, Gary, 36, 46, 76
Herbs and supplements, 189–190
High blood pressure, 37, 78, 210, 255
Higher-level thinking, 46, 50–51, 54–59, 179
High quadrant, 105, 106
Hip rotations, 192
Hirsch-Adlam, Lindsay, 275
Home and work environment, clean, 193–194, 210
Homeostasis, 28
Hydras, 26
Hygiene. *See* Energetic hygiene
Hypertension, 37, 78, 210, 255
Hypnotism, 51
Hypochondria, 33

Illumination technique, 210, 214–215
Immune system, 33, 66
Incense, 193, 204
Indirect clearing methods, 46, 47
Influenza, 252–253
Inner aura, 14, 21
Inner peace, 270
Insomnia, 255–256
Inspirational Breath, 234–235
Integration, state of full, 47–49
Intercostal breathing, 63–64, 74
Internal generation, 142
Invocation, 115, 210
Irritable bowel syndrome, 37, 256

Johns, Tracy, 103
Joint inflammation, 249–250

Karma, 275–278, 282
Kelder, Peter, 221
Kelleher, Maureen, 4
Kilham, Christopher S., 221

Klee, Kenneth, 245
Knee rotations, 192
Kosher Yoga, 77
Krebs cycle, 23
Krieger, Dolores, 11
Kundalini syndrome, 280–281
Kunz, Dora, 11

Lavender oil, 195, 196
Laying on of hands, 12
Leon, Cynthia de, 218
Letting go, 48
Limiting beliefs, 39–41. *See also*
       Negative emotions and lim-
       iting beliefs, clearing
Local Self-Sweeping
       —Chakras, 136–137
       with Colors, 165–167
       —Specific Areas and Joints,
       134–135
Local Sweeping
       of Another Person—Chakras,
       128–130
       of Another Person—Specific
       Areas and Joints, 125–128
Low quadrant, 105
Lung infection, 252–253
Lymph, 66–68
Lymph nodes, 67

Major chakras, 15–17
Mana, 10
Mantras, 69, 193, 204, 209, 215
Martial arts, 11, 68, 185
Martin, Michael, 262
Master Breathing Technique, 77
McCluskey, Moses, 209
Meat, 184–186
Meditation, 30, 47, 68, 69, 199–218
       benefits of, 200–204
       checklist, 217–218
       Dissociation Meditation,
       268–270
       frequency of, 216–217
       general tips, 204–205
       Meditation on Twin Hearts,
       22, 30, 199, 203, 204,

208–216, 270
       Mindfulness Meditation, 30,
       51, 204, 205–208, 270
Memory-Developing Breath
       (Rapid Turtle Breathing),
       226, 232–233
Meng mein (kidneys) chakra, 15,
       17, 19–20, 78, 153, 169,
       171
Menstrual cramps, 159, 256
Mental acuity, sharpened, 201
Mental and physical relaxation, 201
Mentalphysics Exercises, 22, 30,
       220, 222, 231–242
       Cleansing Breath, 238–239
       energy-generating tips, 223–224
       Grand Rejuvenation Breath,
       239–240
       Harmonic Breath (Balancing
       Breathing), 231–232
       Inspirational Breath, 234–235
       Memory-Developing Breath
       (Rapid Turtle Breathing),
       232–233
       Perfection Breath, 236–237
       power of, 222
       Revitalizing Breath, 233–234
       Spiritual Breath, 241–242
       Vibro-Magnetic Breath, 237
Mercy, 277
Meridians, 11, 13, 14, 20–21
Microcosmic orbit, 21
Microwaved food, 185, 186
Middle quadrant, 105
Migraine headaches, 37, 249,
       256–257
Mind, unconscious. *See* Uncon-
       scious mind
Mind-body connection, 33–34
Mindfulness, 48, 49, 202
Mindfulness Meditation, 30, 51,
       204, 205–208, 270
Mini-chakras, 15, 18
Minor chakras, 15, 18
Morning routine, 263

Navel chakra, 15, 17, 19, 78, 149
Neck rotations, 191

Negative emotions, resisting feel-
       ing, 36–37
Negative emotions and limiting
       beliefs, clearing, 29–30,
       45–61, 179
       awareness, 48–49
       direct and indirect methods,
       46–47
       higher-level thinking, 46,
       50–51, 54–59
       integration as goal, 47–49
       pranic breathing and, 70
       self-awareness, 50–54
Negative intrathoracic pressure,
       68
Negative thoughts (persistent),
       257
Neuropeptides, 33–34
Newts, 27

Objectivity, 201–202
O'Connor, Sheevaun, 177
O'Hara, Daniel, 82, 158
OM, 69, 193, 204, 209, 215
Orange prana, 156–158, 160, 161,
       164
Outer aura, 14, 21
Oxygenation, 68

Pain relief (general), 257
Panic attacks, 62
Partial visualization, 134
Perfection Breath, 236–237
Pert, Candace, 33–34
Phobias, 29, 36
Physical exercise, 191–192, 205,
       210
Physiological benefits of pranic
       breathing, 67–68
Plants, scanning, 90–92
Pneumonia, 252–253
Pork, 180, 184–186
Post-surgery routines, 260
Postural conditioning, 65
Potassium, 4
Prana, 10
       colored. *See* Colored pranas

Detecting Your Energetic
Anatomy, 23–25, 84
-generation techniques, 21, 22
principal sources of, 21
stabilizing projected, 145
unconscious mind and, 35
variations in quality of, 21
Pranic anesthesia, 257
Pranic breathing, 30, 47, 51, 59,
62–81, 96, 110, 143, 210.
See also Mentalphysics
Exercises; Tibetan Yogic
Exercises
benefits of, 66–70
checklist, 80–81
notes on, 80
rhythm/retention, 68–69,
78–79
stretching and loosening
diaphragm, 70, 72–74
Pranic Healing. *See also* Self-healing
as adjunct to physician's care,
10
case studies, 1–4, 25–26
colored pranas. *See* Colored
pranas
compared to other types of
energy medicine, 12–14
creation of, 11–12
energetic hygiene. *See* Energetic hygiene
energizing. *See* Energizing
scanning. *See* Scanning
spread of, 12
sweeping. *See* Sweeping
Prayer of St. Francis of Assisi, 212
Pregnant women
colored pranas and, 115, 160,
248
energizing and, 115
sweeping and, 115
Prescription medications, 32, 33
Pre-surgery routines, 259–260
Presweeping Hand Preparation,
116–117
Proper attitude, 272–273, 282
Protection/survival impulse, 35,
38, 40
Psyllium products, 187, 190

Pulse count, 78
Purification, increased, 271, 282

Quarter-squats, 192

Rapid Turtle Breathing, 226,
232–233
Receptors, 33
Red prana, 156–158, 160, 161
Regeneration, 26–27
Reiki, 11–13
Rejuvenation Rite. *See* Tibetan
Yogic Exercises
Relaxation sequence, 52
Repetitive motion injuries, 252
Retention, 68, 69, 78–79
Revitalizing Breath, 233–234
Rhythms, breathing, 68–69, 78–79
Royal jelly, 190

Salamanders, 26–27
Salt, 114, 118, 127, 148, 193,
194–196
bath, 194–195
shower, 195
soap, 195–196
Sarno, John, 37–38
Scanning, 13, 30, 47, 82–109
animals, 92–93
another person, 93–95
checklist, 95–96
Food for Cleanliness and
Energy, 186
General Self-Scanning, 83,
87–90
Hand Sensitivity Exercise 2,
84–87
interpreting results, 105–109
plants, 90–92
Specific Self-Scanning, 98–102
using visualization, 102–105
Schwartz, Jill, 2–3
Second Tibetan Yogic Exercise,
225–226
Sedeno, Elizabeth, 3
Self-awareness, 46, 47, 52–54, 179

Self-Energizing Depleted Areas
or Chakras Using Water
Pump Technique,
151–152
Self-Energizing with Colors—
Stress Relief, 169–171
Self-healing, 245–260
arthritis/joint inflammation,
249–250
asthma, 250
back pain, 250–251
basic laws of, 27–29
burns, 251–252
carpal tunnel, 252
cold, influenza, sinusitis, lung
infection, bronchitis, pneumonia, fever, 252–253
constipation, 253
depression (mild), 253–254
diet and appetite control, 254
earache, 254
energetic hygiene. *See* Energetic hygiene
energy-generation exercises. *See*
Mentalphysics Exercises;
Tibetan Yogic Exercises
energy manipulation. *See* Energizing; Scanning; Sweeping
Experience Form, 289
eyestrain, 254
food poisoning, vomiting or
diarrhea, 255
high blood pressure, 255
insomnia, 255–256
irritable bowel syndrome, 256
meditation. *See* Meditation
menstrual cramps, 256
migraine headaches, 256–257
negative emotions and limiting
beliefs, clearing. *See* Negative emotions and limiting
beliefs, clearing
negative thoughts (persistent),
257
pain relief (general), 257
pranic breathing. *See* Pranic
breathing
pre- and post-surgery routines,
259–260

Self-healing (con't)
   problems associated with,
      247–248
   scientific evidence of energetic
      template, 26–27
   sore throat, 258
   sprains and sports injuries, 258
   stress relief (general), 258
   ulcers, 259
   urinary urgency or frequency,
      251
Self-hypnosis, 48, 68
Self-Sweeping. *See* General Self-
   Sweeping; Local Self-
   Sweeping
Sensitivity, 200
Service, 273–275, 282
Sex chakra, 15, 17–20, 159, 195
Shake in place, 192
Sharpe, Trish, 79
Shoulder rotations, 191
Shu exhalation, 228
Simple Projection: Visualization
   Practice, 146–148
Simultaneous awareness, 208
Single-point concentration, 207
Sinusitis, 252–253
Six Steps Daily Practice Routine,
   60–61, 81, 96, 110, 141,
   154, 175–176, 198, 219,
   242, 260–261
Small heavenly circle, 21
Smith, Elizabeth, 143
Smoking, 63
Solar plexus chakra, 15, 16, 18, 51,
   161, 167, 185, 223
Solar prana, 21, 22, 193, 204
Sore throat, 258
Soul Life, 117
Spallanzani, Lazzaro, 26
Specific Self-Scanning, 83,
   98–102, 110
Spiritual Breath, 241–242
Spiritual cord, pranic breathing
   and, 66, 70
Spiritual development, 271–281
Spiritual restlessness, 269–270
Spleen chakra, 15, 17, 153
Sports injuries, 258

Sprains, 258
Stillness, 202, 209
Stress, 23, 201
Stress relief (general), 258
Sun, as source of prana, 21, 143
Supplements, 189–190
Sweeping, 3, 12, 13, 21, 30, 47,
   111–140. *See also* Self-heal-
   ing
Sweeping (con't)
   basics of, 112–113
   checklist, 137–140
   with colored pranas, 156,
      158–159
   drinking water, 188
   before energizing, 144
   General Self-Sweeping, 130–133
   General Self-Sweeping of
      Health Rays, 133–134
   General Sweeping of Another
      Person, 117–122
   General Sweeping of Health
      Rays of Another Person,
      123–125
   Local Self-Sweeping—
      Chakras, 136–137
   Local Self-Sweeping—Specific
      Areas and Joints, 134–135
   Local Sweeping of Another
      Person—Chakras, 128–130
   Local Sweeping of Another
      Person—Specific Areas and
      Joints, 125–128
   Presweeping Hand Prepara-
      tion, 116–117
   safeguards, 114–115

Tai chi, 11, 205, 220
Taoist systems, 19–21, 142, 275
Tea tree oil, 195
Tension Myofascial Syndrome
   (TMS), 38
Therapeutic Touch, 11–13
Third Tibetan Yogic Exercise,
   226–228
Throat chakra, 15, 16, 18, 19, 149,
   157, 159, 161, 162, 166,
   169, 171, 172

Tibetan Yogic Exercises, 22, 30,
   220, 221, 224–231
   energy-generating tips,
      223–224
   First, 224–225
   Second, 225–226
   Third, 226–228
   Fourth, 228–229
   Fifth, 229–230
Tithing, 278–280, 282
Top quadrant, 105, 106
Torso twists, 192
Traditional Chinese medicine, 11,
   12
Traditional Western scientific
   medicine, 1, 2, 10, 58
Traumatic memories, 29, 35, 37, 41
Trembley, Abraham, 26

Ulcers, 259
Unconscious mind, 34–41, 200,
   208
   clamping down, 37–39
   limiting beliefs, 39–40
   protection/survival impulse,
      35, 38, 40
   reprogramming, 40–41
   resisting feeling negative emo-
      tions, 36–37
United States Pranic Healing
   Center, 285
Unruffling, 13
Urinary urgency or frequency, 37,
   51, 251

Vavra, Naila, 132–133
Vegetables, 184, 185
Ventilation perfusion scan, 64
Vibro-Magnetic Breath, 237
Violet prana, 156, 157, 159, 160,
   164–171
Visualization, 4, 113, 127, 130,
   133, 134, 246. *See also* Col-
   ored pranas; Energizing
   Practice with Colors—Dual
   Colors (Green-Blue),
   163–164

Practice with Colors—Single
    Colors, 162–163
  scanning using, 102–105
Vitamins, 189–190
Vomiting, 255

Washington, Sandra, 209
Waste-removal system, 67–68
Water. *See* Drinking water

Water pump technique, 143. *See
    also* Energizing
  testing pranic flow during,
    171–172
Wheat grass, 190
White blood cells, 9, 10
White prana, 155, 159
Wieczorek, Mark, 209
Wilson, Jason J., 181
Witch hazel, 115, 118

Wrist rolls, 24, 84
Wrist rotations, 192

Yellow prana, 156–158, 160, 161
Yi, 28
Yoga, 12, 20, 68, 142, 220, 280

Zen Buddhism, 48, 201, 202

ABOUT THE AUTHORS

MASTER STEPHEN CO, a personal student of Grandmaster Choa Kok Sui, is one of only four Master Pranic Healers in the world, and the World Pranic Healing Organization's Senior Instructor responsible for teaching throughout the United States. Over the last ten years, Master Co has averaged 100 free, open-to-the-public presentations and instructional classes per year and has taught thousands of people in the United States, Mexico, and the Philippines. He was the first licensee of Pranic Healing outside the Philippines.

ERIC B. ROBINS, M.D, is a board-certified urologist and surgeon in private practice and affiliated with a major hospital in Los Angeles. He received his M.D. degree from Baylor College of Medicine in 1989 and his B.A. in Biology from the University of Texas at Austin. Dr. Robins has received additional training in various alternative healing therapies. He is a certified clinical hypnotherapist, a neurolinguistic programming practitioner, a timeline therapy practitioner, and a certified Pranic Healing instructor.

JOHN MERRYMAN is a freelance writer in Los Angeles. He has been published in *Los Angeles* magazine, *California* magazine, *Cleveland* magazine, and *Orange Coast* magazine, among others. He received his B.A. in English from Kent State University and pursued graduate training in Creative Writing at Ohio State University.